# ALLEN CARR'S
# QUIT DRINKING
## WITHOUT WILLPOWER

SIRIUS

*To Cris Hay—Allen Carr's Easyway to Stop Drinking Alcohol Therapist Extraordinaire.*

This book is based on the principles discovered by Allen Carr through his Easyway method, and developed by him in close collaboration with Robin Hayley, chairman of Allen Carr's Easyway organization and the most senior Allen Carr's Easyway therapist in the world. Having worked closely together across three decades, Allen entrusted Robin with the future development of the Easyway method to insure that his legacy would achieve its full potential.

**SIRIUS**

This edition published in 2023 by Sirius Publishing, a division of Arcturus Publishing Limited,
26/27 Bickels Yard, 151–153 Bermondsey Street,
London SE1 3HA

ISBN: 978-1-78404-541-8
AD001892US

Printed in the US

# ALLEN CARR

Allen Carr was a chain-smoker for over 30 years. In 1983, after countless failed attempts to quit, he went from 100 cigarettes a day to zero without suffering withdrawal pangs, without using willpower, and without putting on weight. He realized that he had discovered what the world had been waiting for—the easy way to stop smoking—and embarked on a mission to help cure the world's smokers.

As a result of the phenomenal success of his method, he gained an international reputation as the world's leading expert on stopping smoking and his network of centers now spans the globe. His first book, *Allen Carr's Easy Way to Stop Smoking*, has sold over 15 million copies, remains a global bestseller, and has been published in over forty different languages. Hundreds of thousands of smokers have successfully quit at Allen Carr's Easyway Centers where, with a success rate of over 90 percent, they guarantee you'll find it easy to stop or your money back.

Allen Carr's Easyway method has been successfully applied to a host of issues including weight control, alcohol, and other addictions and fears. A list of Allen Carr centers appears at the back of this book. If you require any assistance or if you have any questions, please do not hesitate to contact your nearest center.

For more information about Allen Carr's Easyway, please visit **www.allencarr.com**

# Allen Carr's Easyway

## The key that will set you free

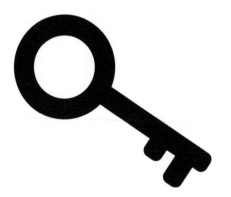

# CONTENTS

# INTRODUCTION

The five hours I spent in a session with Allen Carr at his center in London over 25 years ago changed my life. I entered that session as an addict who had to know when I could have my next fix or I would panic; who was convinced that I would have to give up one of life's pleasures and would feel miserable and deprived; who was frightened that I wouldn't be able to deal with stress; and who found it almost impossible to imagine a life without my drug. I left with no need or desire to continue taking the drug. I suffered no withdrawal pangs. Like others I knew who had seen Allen, I found it easy to stop. It took no willpower. There was no feeling of deprivation; instead I felt huge relief and utter elation that I was free. It was truly extraordinary.

The drug I was addicted to was nicotine, but I realized at once that Allen Carr had devised a method that could help any addict quit easily and immediately, and I wrote to him asking if I could join him in his mission. It was my great good fortune that I was accepted. Allen then trained me as a therapist and we set up the second center together in Birmingham. Shortly afterward I was lucky enough to be appointed Managing Director of a company formed to spread the method all over the world and my vision of a global organization began to become a reality.

Today, more than 400,000 people have visited our centers in over 50 countries around the world. The centers still provide a full and genuine money-back guarantee on demand, if you do not stop for at least three months. Most people require just one session. Fewer than 10 percent of all those who have attended the centers have claimed their money back.

In addition, Allen Carr's Easyway books have sold more than 20 million copies, been translated into 40 languages, and read by an estimated 50 million people in 57 different countries.

This phenomenal success has been achieved not through advertising or marketing but through the personal recommendations of the millions of happy ex-addicts who've quit with the method. Allen Carr's Easyway has spread all over the world for one reason alone: BECAUSE IT WORKS.

*Quit Drinking Without Willpower* applies Allen's now world-famous method to the most commonly consumed addictive drug of all: alcohol. The method does not preach nor does it state the obvious. Drinkers know it's bad for their health and costing them a fortune. The worst thing though is the slavery, the feeling of being controlled. Perhaps you've tried to quit before by using willpower, by going to Alcoholics Anonymous, or by trying hypnosis, acupuncture, laser therapy, or some other gimmick. The chances are that you felt deprived and miserable and ended up failing. Perhaps you fear that you will never be able to enjoy meals or social occasions without a drink and that you will be unable to cope with stress. Perhaps you also dread the trauma you suffered on previous failed attempts and fear you can never get free from the craving.

Easyway is different. This book is the key that will set you free from this prison. It will completely change your mindset by stripping away all the illusions and fears that have kept you trapped. Easyway does not involve willpower or deprivation as it removes the desire to drink and you will be able to look forward to enjoying social occasions more and handling stress better right from the moment you become a nondrinker.

Allen Carr's Easyway transformed my life. It can do the same for you.

Robin Hayley M.A. (Oxon), M.B.A., M.A.A.C.T.I.
Chairman, Allen Carr's Easyway (International) Ltd

# Chapter 1

# THE KEY

## IN THIS CHAPTER

*MY CLAIM  *A METHOD THAT WORKS  *ARE YOU AN ALCOHOLIC?
*COMMON MISCONCEPTIONS  *NO LAUGHING MATTER  *YOU'RE
NOT ALONE  *WAITING FOR A MIRACLE  *THE INSTRUCTIONS

*This book will enable you to stop drinking immediately, painlessly, and permanently, without any sense of deprivation or sacrifice. What's more, you will not need to use willpower. You will find it easy.*

Does that sound too good to be true? A permanent end to your drinking problem that requires no willpower, pain, or sacrifice? Until now, everything you will have been told about problem drinking will have led you to believe that this claim cannot possibly be true. And yet you've decided to give it a try for one very good reason: You desperately want it to be true. You're sick and tired of being a slave to drink, of wanting to stop but finding yourself powerless to do so, and every other method you've tried has failed you. Your decision could be the most important one you've ever made in your life. I promise you that it's absolutely possible to free yourself from alcohol, regardless of who you are or what your personal circumstances may be. In fact, provided you follow the right method, it's more than just possible—it's guaranteed.

A lot of drinkers who come to our centers do so with the support and encouragement of a friend or family member. This book will act as your friend, as well as your instructor, as you make the wonderful journey out of the alcohol trap. Like any true friend, it will not judge you or embarrass you, nor will it put pressure on you to do anything you don't want to do. All I ask is that you remain honest about your desire to stop, keep an open mind, and follow the instructions. Do that and you cannot fail to escape the misery of the prison in which alcohol has trapped you. It's that easy.

People think it's hard to quit because that's what we're told. Whether it comes from the medical profession, other drinkers who have tried to quit, or organizations like Alcoholics Anonymous, the message is always the same: Quitting is hard.

With this method you will come to see the beautiful truth that escaping from the trap you find yourself in can be easy and enjoyable. You do not need to suffer the misery caused by drinking, nor do you need to suffer in order to get free. You can quit drinking and regain control of your life simply by doing just two things:

1.  Understanding the nature of the problem.

2.  Following an effective method to solve it.

This book will enable you to do both by tackling your drinking problem with the most successful method ever designed for overcoming addiction.

You may have already had your final drink. Some people vow never to drink again before they start reading this book, but others continue to drink right up until the last instruction. You can carry on drinking as you wish until you reach the end of the book, but it's recommended that you only read this book while sober, otherwise you will not fully take in what you're reading. It's also crucial by the end of the book that you're left in no doubt about never wanting to drink again.

## A DRINK TOO FAR

Alcoholics Anonymous is a fine organization staffed by well-meaning people with some excellent ideas. One of the questions they ask concerns the drink that tips you over the edge, from controlled drinking into drunkenness. Is it the third? The fifth? The tenth maybe? Everyone gives a different answer, but there is only one correct answer and it applies to everybody: It's the first drink that's the problem. AA are spot on in pointing out the simple truth that if you never took the first drink, you simply could not have an alcohol problem. So the first drink is the one to avoid.

Until I applied my method to the problem, there were two approaches to getting drinking under control:

1.   The willpower method.

2.   The Alcoholics Anonymous approach.

Both methods focus on the temptation to drink. With the willpower method, you're told that you have to fight the temptation. People who try this feel deprived and miserable and the majority go back to drinking sooner or later. In due course I will explain in greater detail exactly why the willpower method doesn't work.

Alcoholics Anonymous tells you that you have to rise above the temptation to drink. The problem with this approach is that, as with the willpower method, it means you have to live with the temptation for the rest of your life. As long as you have the temptation in your life, you will be vulnerable.

The good news is there is another way—a method that has successfully cured millions of people of addictions to drinking, smoking, and other drugs, as well as overeating, overspending and gambling:

3.   Allen Carr's Easyway.

With Easyway, the desire to drink is removed altogether. Therefore, the temptation and vulnerability that haunt you with methods 1 and 2 are eradicated.

## THE "ALCOHOLIC" STIGMA

Many of the drinkers who come to our centers saying they need help to stop drinking for one reason or another balk at the term "alcoholic." Their idea of an alcoholic is often a disheveled, shambolic drunkard, who reeks of booze and is incapable of lucid thought or conversation. But our clients are nothing like that when we meet them. In fact, in most cases they conceal their drinking problem incredibly well.

Why do they conceal it? Because they fear the stigma. Society is intolerant of those it calls alcoholics. In fact, society's attitude to alcohol is riddled with contradictions. Alcohol is a drug, nobody disputes that, but while all other so-called recreational drugs (including, increasingly, smoking) are marginalized or criminalized, for some reason alcohol is embraced as not only socially acceptable but as a social necessity. Try throwing a party without booze!

As soon as we're old enough to drink legally in public (and often before), adults take great joy in buying us our first alcoholic drinks, encouraging us to force down those first repulsive sips, and "develop a taste for it." They laugh knowingly when we feel awful afterward, and when it comes to celebrating, how do they go about it? Champagne!

And yet when the woman next door starts smelling of booze; when you see her smashed at one party after another; when she asks to borrow money and you know she's lying about what she needs it for; when she's spotted drinking on a bench in the park; when she fails to turn up at school to collect her kids; how does society react? With tut-tutting, shaking of the head, and disapproving whispers of "How could she be so irresponsible?"

The general assumption is that alcoholics have only themselves to blame, that they're weak or self-indulgent, and that it's their fault for failing to control their drinking. No wonder people with a drink problem tend to do their utmost to hide it. Unfortunately this only makes the problem worse because in hiding it from society, we also hide it from ourselves. We deny that we have a problem and thereby deny ourselves the opportunity to solve it.

Let's get one thing straight: Addiction to alcohol is not a weakness. It's something that can happen to anyone, rich or poor, strong-willed or weak-willed, intelligent or stupid. The reason society thinks it's a weakness is because we're all fooled into believing that "normal" drinkers are in control. As you will discover by reading this book, no drinker is really in control.

If you don't want to call yourself an alcoholic, that's fine. What you call the problem is not important; what's essential is that you acknowledge that your alcohol consumption is out of control. Why else would you be reading this book?

## COMMON MISCONCEPTIONS

The myth that alcoholics are weak is just one of the misconceptions that cloud the issue of drinking. Here are some others:

**Problem drinking means drinking every day.**
Frequency varies among problem drinkers. Some drink only on weekends, others feel they have to have a drink as soon as they

wake up. The effects can be devastating in either case.

**Problem drinkers are driven to it by difficult circumstances.**
Anyone can fall into the alcohol trap. Problem drinkers from all walks of life tend to blame their circumstances, or other people, in order to rationalize their behavior, but there's only one true cause: alcohol addiction.

**Poor people are more prone to become problem drinkers.**
Everyone is susceptible to the drinking trap, no matter how rich or poor they are. Millions of wealthy people fall victim to alcohol addiction and although they may generally buy more expensive drinks, they will drink anything that's available if necessary to try to satisfy their craving.

It doesn't matter who you are, when you started drinking, how often or how much, you do so for the same reason: to get the alcohol.

### IN HIS OWN WORDS: DAVID

I had a job that I loved, but I was forced to retire. I'd never been a drinker before, but losing my job hit me badly and I was bored having nothing to do, so I started going to the pub.

The drinking just took me over. I'd go on binges that lasted for days. It shattered my family and I ended up losing my marriage. I hurt so many people and the stupid thing is I can honestly say I didn't even like it.

I used alcohol to try to fill a gap in my life. I didn't expect it to replace an interesting, meaningful job, but I believed it could make my situation more bearable. I was wrong; it just made everything worse. But because I came to feel that it was my only escape, the worse things got, the more I drank. Even though I knew it was killing me, I just couldn't see a way out. I never realized then that it was alcohol itself that was dragging me further and further down.

## NO LAUGHING MATTER

Problem drinking is a devastating condition. It causes severe anxiety, illness, other addictions, the breakdown of relationships, loss of employment, financial ruin, and even death.

### *IN THE U.K. ALCOHOL PLAYS A PART IN:*

44% of all violent crime
42% of domestic violence
80% of road deaths on Friday nights
20% of murders

These numbers concern only the physical violence that results from alcohol. They are in addition to the other destructive effects mentioned previously. Nevertheless, the figures speak for themselves: The damage caused by this drug is out of control.

It seems reasonable to assume from the fact that you're reading this book that you do not feel in control of your drinking. A lot of people who come to us say they're bored with drinking, but they just can't seem to stop. They sense that drinking gives them no real pleasure, yet they continue to do it. They've tried to quit and found they couldn't. No matter how hard they tried, their willpower eventually gave out and they fell back into drinking. As a result, they feel weak-willed and stupid and they can't understand why they're powerless to stop.

The fact is

### *YOU ARE NOT POWERLESS AND*
### *YOU DON'T LACK WILLPOWER*

In fact heavy drinkers tend to be rather strong-willed for reasons I'll explain later. Allen Carr's Easyway doesn't involve willpower in any case. It will enable you to see the truth about alcohol addiction, and once you understand you will find it easy to stop.

### YOU'RE NOT ALONE

No matter how lonely you may feel with your drinking problem, you're not alone. The World Health Organization estimates that there are 140 million alcoholics in the world today.

It's important to realize that your drinking problem is not

unique to you. There is nothing about your personal situation that makes alcohol addiction inevitable. Despite the fact that problem drinkers often succumb to other addictions, such as smoking or gambling, this should not be taken as an indication that certain types of people are susceptible to addiction. If you think that might be the reason for your problem, please put that thought out of your mind at once. As I will explain in the coming chapters, alcoholism is a human problem that has nothing to do with the way we, as individuals, are made, but is the result of a subtle chemical addiction compounded by massive brainwashing about what alcohol does for you.

Whoever you are, whatever you do, wherever you live, however much money you earn, you can find yourself a slave to alcohol. The good news is that there is an easy way to escape from the prison and you are holding it in your hands right now.

## WAITING FOR A MIRACLE

**"I knew I needed help, but I still didn't want to stop."**

This statement encapsulates the tug-of-war all problem drinkers battle with. You know it's causing you misery and damaging your life, yet you feel compelled to go on doing it. The misery gets worse, yet the compulsion to go on drinking only gets stronger. You really want to quit, yet at the same time you're terrified of even trying.

This emotional tug-of-war leaves you feeling confused and trapped. Whichever way you turn, the doors close on you. At the same time, you're aware that your drinking is having an impact on those around you. You try to conceal it from them, in the hope that one day a miracle will happen and you'll wake free from the nightmare.

But you can only keep a drinking problem secret for a limited time. Because of the effect it has on you mentally and physically, the outward signs become obvious to anyone who knows you. The futility of even trying to keep a lid on the problem often leads to a "Devil may care" attitude. "I can't do anything about it so what's the point of pretending?"

It's heartbreaking to watch someone you care about falling into the alcohol trap. As in David's case, no matter how much somebody loves you, there's only so much drunken behavior they can put up with. At some point they will decide they've had enough and leave. And once you lose the people who care about you and you find yourself alone, the tendency is to cling ever more tightly to the thing that's destroying you in the mistaken belief that it's your last pleasure or crutch.

Let me make one thing very clear from the start: I'm not here to scare you. That is not how this method works. If scare tactics worked, I would have no hesitation in using them. The fact is that every problem drinker is well aware of the powerful reasons not to drink and yet they go on doing it. However, you do need to be aware of the facts about alcohol, because it's the misconceptions that prevent us from getting free. Alcohol is an addictive poison that destroys your health, wealth, and happiness and shortens your life. Added to that, the misery of addiction often leads to other addictions, such as smoking, other drugs, gambling, and overeating.

Some alcoholics consciously drink themselves to death. The realization that you're not, in fact, in control of your drinking—that in fact it is the drinking which controls you—can ultimately lead to despair. Most drinkers, however, maintain the will to survive. They go on enduring the misery, day after day, feeling helpless to do anything about it, and just waiting for the day when some miracle occurs and they find they're no longer hooked on booze. If that's you, I have good news for you:

## *YOU DON'T NEED A MIRACLE*

The solution is in your hands. Perhaps you're afraid that I'm going to ask you to carry out a series of grueling tasks in order to get free. On the contrary, this method not only makes it easy to quit, but you can even enjoy the process right from the start.

In fact in order to quit, you don't actually have to do anything. All you have not to do is take another drink. It's easy, provided you change the way you think about alcohol. This method strips away the brainwashing that makes us believe that stopping involves sacrifice and deprivation and replaces it with the truth. Once you understand and accept the truth, you can then follow some simple steps and become a happy nondrinker.

As you read through the book, I will give you a series of instructions. These instructions are very simple and if you follow them all, you cannot fail to solve your drink problem. The first instruction is:

## *FOLLOW ALL THE INSTRUCTIONS*

Easyway works like the combination to a safe. If you know the combination and you apply the numbers in the correct order, the lock springs and the door swings open. But if you're missing any of the numbers, or you apply them in the wrong order, the door will remain locked.

I ask you, therefore, to follow the method exactly as it's set out. Take each instruction and apply it in order. Resist the temptation to skip ahead or you will miss a crucial part of the combination. Remember, at the end of this book lies your liberation from the tyranny of alcohol. I fully understand that you want to get to that point as quickly as possible and I sympathize, but please be patient. The method works—that has been proven millions of times over throughout the world—and it will work for you, provided you follow all the instructions.

## SUMMARY

- Whatever methods you've tried to quit with so far have not worked for you, but this one will.
- You don't control alcohol, alcohol controls you.
- You're not alone and your drinking problem has nothing to do with your genetic makeup or character.
- You don't need a miracle.
- Follow all the instructions.

# Chapter 2

# PERCEPTION AND PRECONCEPTION

## IN THIS CHAPTER

• *WHY WE DON'T JUST STOP* • *TRYING AND FAILING*
• *WILLPOWER* • *THE MYTH OF THE CHARMING ADDICT*
• *DENIAL* • *HOW QUITTING CAN BE EASY*

*Why do we find it so hard to stop drinking even when we know it's ruining our life?*

Many of the people who come to our centers with an alcohol problem say they've grown bored with drinking. They sense it's making them miserable and they desperately want to quit.

Moving bricks from one pile to another is pretty boring. If I asked you to move a pile of bricks just for the sake of it, and offered you nothing in return, would you do it? Of course not. You would tell me not to be absurd. So why don't drinkers who have become bored with drinking just stop?

The reason lies in the way our brains are wired. While our rational mind may tell us that drinking is causing us untold harm and that we must stop, our addicted mind continues to harbor a desire to drink. Why? Because it has been conditioned to believe that drinking alcohol gives us some sort of pleasure or support. In order to break free from this tug-of-war and allow our rational minds to regain control, we must undo the brainwashing that causes the desire to drink.

Before we can begin to remove the brainwashing, it's essential that you recognize and accept that you have been brainwashed and take a positive attitude to escaping from the trap. This is what drinkers who try to stop on the willpower method find incredibly hard to do and that is why they usually end up remaining in the trap.

I called my method Easyway because it provided smokers with an easy way to quit. The same method has worked successfully for people with other addictions, including alcohol and other drugs, gambling, overspending, and overeating. One major difference between Easyway and all the other methods that claim to help overcome addiction is that the other methods begin with the message that it will not be easy. This in itself is another piece of brainwashing that keeps addicts in the trap, because the harder you think quitting is going to be, the more fearful you will be of trying, the more you will put off your attempt and the more you will seek refuge in what you feel is your last little crutch.

## THE BELIEF THAT QUITTING WILL BE HARD KEEPS DRINKERS IN THE ALCOHOL TRAP

Remember the claim I made at the start:

*This book will enable you to stop drinking immediately, painlessly, and permanently, without the need for willpower or feeling any sense of deprivation or sacrifice. You will find it easy.*

Perhaps you're thinking, "If this method actually makes it easy to quit drinking, why doesn't everyone use it?" It's a perfectly understandable question and one that most of our successful quitters have asked at one time or another. It's important that you're skeptical. I want you to question everything you've ever been told about alcohol and drinking. By questioning things, you will arrive at the truth. The problem is that most people never question the assumptions society has about alcohol, and so they are passed from generation to generation.

I can assure you Easyway works. Millions of ex-addicts around the world can vouch for that. But I don't expect you simply to believe me. In fact, at this stage it doesn't matter if you believe me or not, what's important is that you follow the instructions. What have you got to lose? Unless you make the attempt to stop, you're in for more of the same misery, further deterioration in your physical and mental health, and the prospect of remaining a slave for the rest of your life.

Let's examine the reasons why you believe that quitting will be hard.

## PROVEN FAILURES

You probably know of other drinkers, or people with other addictions such as smoking or gambling, who have tried to quit but failed. Perhaps you have tried yourself but been pulled back into the trap by a force that was too strong for you to resist.

Every failed attempt to quit an addiction is a big setback. Your self-esteem, which is already low because of the helplessness you feel as an addict, takes a further battering. You see your failure as a reflection on yourself and regard yourself as pathetic, weak, and inferior to all those people who appear to sail through life without such problems. At the same time, you reinforce the impression that your addiction is a prison from which you will never have the strength to escape.

And it's not only the person who tries and fails to quit who is affected by each failure. Every time we hear of someone else who has made an attempt to stop but failed, it reinforces our belief that stopping must be incredibly difficult. When we look at these people, and even when we look at ourselves, we see people who are, in many ways, strong. People don't become addicts because they're weak. Many highly intelligent, single-minded, brave, and strong people suffer the misery of addiction and find it impossible to escape for the simple reason that they're going about it the wrong way.

## LOSING THE WILL

I began by saying that in order to overcome your drink problem you must take a positive attitude to escaping from the trap. You may have interpreted that to mean that you need to be strong-willed. Many people make this assumption, but it's false and can result in the addict remaining in the trap for the rest of their life.

It's essential that you understand that you do not need willpower to overcome your addiction. People who try to stop and fail usually assume it's because they lack willpower. They believe that it must be some weakness in them that prevents them from succeeding.

This is another aspect of the brainwashing. It's a misconception perpetuated even by the "help" organizations that claim to help us quit. Easyway is the one method that does not tell you to use willpower. It also happens to be the most effective method ever devised.

I said that this book will help you to overcome your drink problem painlessly and easily. When you reach the end and experience the elation of becoming free, you will know exactly what I mean. Right now, however, you may still be finding it hard to believe that it's possible to stop without applying immense reserves of willpower and going through a period of trauma. Believe me, it is possible.

You have a choice: You can choose to keep reading, follow the instructions, and see if I'm right, or you can choose to continue the way you're going now, suffering the misery of alcohol addiction, falling deeper and deeper into the pit, losing money, friends, possessions and self-respect, and coming ever closer to the point where you can see no point in living.

If you think you've failed to quit in the past because you lack the willpower, I have nothing but good news. You don't need willpower. You failed to quit because you were using a method that doesn't work. By picking up this book, you have embarked on a method that has been proven to work for millions of people all over the world. What's more, it makes it easy.

## WHAT AM I WITHOUT BOOZE?

In addition to the false belief that quitting has to be hard, some people believe that by "giving up the booze" they will lose a valuable part of their identity. This just shows how addiction can twist our judgement. Despite the misery, the slavery, the ill health, the torment, the loss of self-respect, and all the other damage caused by alcohol, some drinkers continue to see drinking as something that makes them somehow attractive.

Alcohol is widely perceived as a "sociable" drug and most drinkers are under the misconception that they become more interesting, more witty, and more fun when they've had a drink. But that's not the issue here. There is something in the self-destruction of the drinker that is sometimes portrayed as attractive.

No one wants to be considered "safe." The word implies boring, unadventurous, predictable. We prefer to be seen as a bit "dangerous"—i.e. exciting, unpredictable, never dull. In books and movies we tend to feel intimidated by characters who show no vulnerability and we warm to the ones who are flawed. The shambolic character who battles through life against his own demons, be it drink, other drugs, gambling, or whatever, usually wins our sympathy and affection over the one who appears to be in complete control and never puts a foot wrong.

We're fed these stereotypes time and time again through movies, TV, literature, and other media, and so it's hardly surprising that our own self-image often appears more attractive if there are obvious flaws. If we take the alcohol problem out of our life, will we lose what we perceive to be our "charm" or "charisma?"

But wait a minute. Isn't it true that you spend most of your time trying to conceal the fact that you have a drink problem?

If your flaws are so charming, why do you keep covering

them up? Why not flaunt them for the world to see?

Of course, the reason we don't do that is because we're ashamed of the way drinking affects us. Alcohol also has a serious effect on mental health, leading to conditions such as anxiety, depression, neurosis, paranoia, and dementia. We don't want everybody to know that we have lost control, that we've lost the ability to enjoy life, and that we're stuck in a trap from which we feel incapable of escape.

There is nothing charming about being addicted to alcohol. Next time some incoherent drunken stranger starts blubbering embarrassingly in your face, or you're the target of unwanted drunken advances from the opposite sex, or you see a drunkard turning nasty or violent because of alcohol, ask yourself how attractive that is.

Of course, the effects on your physical health are also devastating. Cirrhosis of the liver is the condition most commonly associated with excessive drinking, but alcohol can cause a number of other conditions that are anything but charming, including stomach ulcers, pancreatitis, gastritis, and impotence, as well as high blood pressure, strokes, and cancer.

So if you feel that you will be a less appealing character without alcohol in your life, think again!

### IN HIS OWN WORDS: SEAN

My father died when I was 22 from cirrhosis of the liver. I watched his deterioration, the agony he went through, the ravings, and ultimately the ruptured vein that led to him dying in a pool of his own blood and vomit. I couldn't imagine a worse way to go, but by the time he died I was already well on my way to becoming an alcoholic myself.

My dad had been sick through his drinking for many years and yet that still didn't stop me from going down the same path. In fact, I think it must have played a part in my own addiction. Perhaps I couldn't see any other way in life. This was my lot. I was a drinker.

I had numerous health scares and after each one I would come off the booze for a few weeks or even months. But I would always go back to it again. I just couldn't see myself living without alcohol.

I somehow made it to the age of 40 and celebrated my birthday by going on a binge that lasted ten days. I woke up in the hospital, covered in sweat, with a throbbing ache in my stomach and a splitting headache.

When I saw my yellow skin I recognized the signs from seeing my dad go through the same nightmare. I was told I had acute alcoholic hepatitis but I was lucky—my liver still had a chance, provided I stopped drinking for good. I was also informed that I had fallen down a flight of stairs and fractured my skull. I was lucky to be alive.

It was the wake-up call I needed. Something

struck a chord in my head, telling me I didn't have to go the same way as my dad. I had a choice. I had always assumed that alcohol addiction was my lot in life, but I quit with Allen Carr's Easyway three years ago and I don't miss it at all.

## DENIAL

Everyone with a drink problem wishes they could quit. The fact that they feel incapable of doing so makes them feel foolish and weak, and so they try to make themselves feel better by concocting excuses for why they continue to drink.

"I like the taste."

"It helps me unwind."

"I just do it to be sociable."

These are all examples of how drinkers delude themselves. They imply that the drinker has made a controlled choice to drink in each case. But as everyone with a drink problem knows deep down:

### *YOU DON'T CONTROL ALCOHOL, ALCOHOL CONTROLS YOU*

However, many drinkers are afraid to admit this fact. They make up excuses for why they drink because they're afraid to accept the real reason: they're in a trap—a trap called alcohol addiction.

This is frightening for a drinker to admit because it forces them to face their options: stay in the trap and continue to suffer the misery, or try to escape. Escaping seems more frightening than staying in because they have been brainwashed into believing it will be a difficult, painful ordeal and that they will spend the rest of their life feeling deprived. Faced with that prospect, they tend to put off the "evil day" indefinitely.

But when you realize that escaping need be neither painful nor difficult, and that life immediately becomes more enjoyable without alcohol, the situation changes completely. Rather than facing two evils, you find yourself facing one evil and one easy, happy option. Who in their right mind would choose the former?

## THE EASY OPTION

We've established what will happen if you continue to drink. Now let's contemplate the life that awaits you as a happy nondrinker.

### Health

Drinking affects your health both mentally and physically. In addition to the medical conditions already mentioned, it affects the way you take care of yourself. For example, you neglect your nutritional needs and abuse your body with junk food, or sometimes no food at all. Sleep also suffers. When you're free from the alcohol trap, you will enjoy eating well, sleeping soundly, and generally feeling a fantastic glow of health and happiness.

### Control

With your life back under your control, you will be able to make plans that will leave you feeling happy and fulfilled. You will be in control of your behavior and your destiny.

### Honesty

Without your addiction, you will no longer feel the need to cover your tracks, conceal what you're up to, lie to your loved ones, or take money dishonestly to fund your addiction. As a result you will feel far less stressed and angry.

### Self-respect

Your behavior towards others and the realization that you're no longer a slave to alcohol will make you feel much better about yourself. Every time you think about your achievement in escaping the alcohol trap, you will feel a burst of elation and pride.

### Time

When you no longer spend your life focusing on your next drink, you will find you have so much more time to pursue things that you will find genuinely rewarding.

### Money

Think of the money you will save. On average we spend around $100,000 on alcohol in a lifetime. For problem drinkers the figure is a lot higher than that; it can easily be over $400,000. Think of the genuine fun you could have with that money.

All these wonderful benefits await you when you escape the

alcohol trap. In order to do that, you don't need willpower, nor do you need to suffer or feel deprived. All you need to do is unravel the illusions that have put you in the trap in the first place and then you'll find it easy. In fact you can even enjoy the process.

How do you know that what I say is true and not just another piece of brainwashing? I will make that clear in the coming chapters; for now I ask you only to accept that what I say could be true and this is my second instruction:

### *KEEP AN OPEN MIND*

You may already regard yourself as an open-minded person, but we tend to go through life with our minds largely made up by other people.

For example, when you see the sun rise in the morning, you interpret it as a ball of fiery gases burning millions of miles away, which has the appearance of rising in the sky because the Earth is spinning. How do you know that's the case? Because you've been presented with some very convincing arguments by people with expertise in that field, none of whom have yet contradicted the theory, and the explanation tallies with what you see. Not so long ago, people believed that it was actually God driving a fiery chariot across the sky. That was the explanation put forward by the learned men of the time and it tallied with what people saw.

Now take a look at the two tables on the next page, one square, one rectangular.

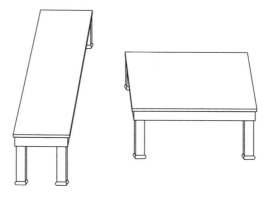

If I were to tell you that the dimensions of each table are exactly the same, you'd be extremely skeptical, wouldn't you? You've already accepted that it's one square table and one rectangular one because that's what I told you it is and it tallies with what you see.

However, the fact is they're both identical. If you don't believe me, take a ruler and measure them. Extraordinary, isn't it?

The reason I'm showing you this illusion is because I want to demonstrate how our minds can easily be tricked into accepting as true something that is false.

When you started drinking you believed that you were doing so out of choice, but what if you were basing your choice on false information?

As you read this book, I want you to remember these tables and keep an open mind, so that even if I tell you something that you find difficult to believe, you will accept the possibility that what I say is true.

## SUMMARY

- We are brainwashed into believing we can't enjoy life without alcohol.

- Failing to quit by using willpower reinforces the illusion that it has to be difficult.

- You don't need willpower to become free.

- There's nothing attractive about problem drinking.

- Addicts lie to themselves to cover up the real reason why they drink.

- Think of all the wonderful gains you'll make by quitting.

- Keep an open mind.

Chapter 3

# FIRST STEPS TO FREEDOM

*Your escape from the alcohol trap has already begun. Our job now is to remove the brainwashing that causes your desire to drink.*

There was a time when I was just like Sean, resigned to an early death through a habit I just couldn't seem to kick. My problem was smoking. I'd watched it kill my father and I assumed the same fate lay in store for me. I tried and failed to quit on numerous occasions but I just couldn't rid myself of my craving for cigarettes.

Sometimes I managed to go without for months, but I always went back to it eventually, like a man struggling to claw his way out of a slippery pit and, just when he thinks he's nearly out, losing his grip and sliding back in. It was as if there were some unseen force pulling me down.

Then something happened that, like a miracle, enabled me to escape immediately. It wasn't a miracle, it was a chance comment that made me realize my smoking was not a habit but an addiction.

That was the unseen force that was dragging me back into the pit time after time, and as soon as I understood that, I was able to conquer it immediately and permanently. Why? Because it changed my whole way of looking at the problem.

Until then I had believed that smoking was just a habit, albeit a particularly nasty one, that I couldn't seem to give up. I assumed that it must do something for me, otherwise why couldn't I just stop? After all, I had powerful reasons for quitting: the bad health, the cost, the smell, the despair of my family.

The mistake I was making was in trying to find a logical reason why I smoked. I was unaware that the drug had twisted my logic. Once I recognized my smoking problem as drug addiction, I was able to understand the nature of the trap.

## WHAT IS ADDICTION?

The word "addiction", like "alcoholic," is one that most people do not wish to hear applied to themselves. You will have noticed that I've used it several times already in this book and it may have caused you some alarm. Perhaps your view of an addict is the miserable junkie, curled up in the corner, out of his head on some drug, or shaking and desperate because he can't get a fix. Funnily enough, I used to get like that when I ran out of cigarettes and I've seen plenty of drinkers who fit that description when they're desperate for a drink. But addiction is not a word to shy away from. For me it was the key to getting free, because it opened my eyes to two crucial facts about my inability to quit smoking:

1. It was not a weakness in my character.

2. It was not some magical quality in the cigarette.

Both these beliefs had left me feeling powerless to quit. Recognizing that my problem was drug addiction enabled me to follow the simple steps to escape.

My addiction was smoking, but all addictions work in the same way. The effect of the drug replaces your natural coping mechanisms, so you turn more and more to the drug for support and feel less and less able to cope without it. Not all addictions involve a drug like alcohol or nicotine. Gambling, for example, is an addiction whereby the "drug" of betting money causes the same psychological feeling of dependency that I've just described. As you fall deeper and deeper into the trap, it becomes harder and harder to see a way out.

## *ADDICTION BLINDS YOU TO REALITY*

Feeling unable to stop drinking despite the harm you know it's causing you is a sure sign of addiction. As with all addictions, it's the illusion that the drug provides a genuine pleasure or support that keeps you trapped. Drinkers suffer the illusion that alcohol helps them relax, gives them courage, makes them more eloquent, and fun to be with. In fact, it does the complete opposite.

As the alcohol leaves your body, you start to feel uptight. There are effective ways to relieve stress, but as a society of drinkers we're at a disadvantage: We have been brainwashed to believe that alcohol does the job. So instead of doing something genuinely relaxing, we do the one thing that will guarantee we end up more stressed: we have another drink. And so a vicious circle is formed.

### *WHAT WE INTERPRET AS PLEASURE FROM THE DRUG IS IN FACT RELIEF FROM WITHDRAWAL*

Drinking temporarily relieves the uncomfortable feeling of the body withdrawing from alcohol—a feeling that nondrinkers do not suffer from in the first place. Therefore,

### *DRINKERS DRINK IN ORDER TO FEEL LIKE NONDRINKERS!*

When you understand and accept the simple truth that drinking does absolutely nothing for you whatsoever, you will realize that stopping, therefore, involves no sacrifice or deprivation and you will find it easy to do so.

### HOW EASYWAY WORKS

Every drinker who picks up this book is eager to discover the secret of this magical cure to their alcohol problem and probably wonders why I don't just come out with it in Chapter 1, but I hope by now you're beginning to see the two fallacies in this expectation:

1. It's not a secret.

2. There's no magic.

Easyway is a method that works by applying undisputable logic to strip away the brainwashing that keeps us in the alcohol trap, and replace it with understanding, thereby removing your desire to drink. The key is made up of the instructions I give you throughout the book and, as I explained in Chapter 1, it must be used like the combination lock of a safe. Each instruction must be understood and applied in order for the combination to work.

I have already given you the first two instructions and in getting this far you have taken your first steps to freedom, but please be patient. The key to your escape does not lie in the final chapter or the first chapter, or any chapter alone; the whole book is the key.

The key works by removing the illusion that you are making a sacrifice by stopping. In order to do that, we need to change your frame of mind. So let's identify what's wrong with your current frame of mind as a drinker, remove that from your way of thinking and let logic and reason undo the brainwashing you've been subjected to ever since you were a child.

### EVER-PRESENT DANGER

An alcohol addict is caught in a trap, just like someone who's stepped on a mantrap. Between us we have the two things we need to set him free: he contributes a strong desire to be released and I have the key that will release him. All he has to do is follow my instructions.

However, once he's released there is another danger: The trap still exists and we have to insure that he does not walk into it again.

## LET'S MAKE IT PERMANENT

People with addictions like drinking, smoking, and gambling are notorious for "giving up" and starting again, so helping you to escape from the trap is the first step. The second is insuring you never walk into it again. We can do this by making sure you understand the nature of the trap.

Unlike a mantrap, the alcohol trap is essentially psychological. It exists only in the mind—an illusion conjured up by a combination of the chemical addiction and massive brainwashing. Like the table illusion in the last chapter, you have been fed a false view of reality, which has created the illusion that you get a genuine pleasure or support from drinking and that quitting will involve pain and sacrifice. But after seeing those tables, you should now be open to the possibility that those beliefs are false.

It's also worth bearing in mind that 10 percent of adults have lived their lives without ever falling for the alcohol trap, despite being subjected to a massive amount of brainwashing. This brings us to the real difference between drinkers and nondrinkers. Obviously one drinks and the other doesn't, but that's not the whole story.

## THE CRUCIAL DIFFERENCE BETWEEN DRINKERS AND NONDRINKERS IS THAT THE LATTER HAVE NO DESIRE TO DRINK

No one forces you to drink. No one holds a gun to your head. You find the drink, you pour it, you bring the glass to your lips. The fact that part of your brain wishes you didn't, or can't understand why you do, doesn't change the situation.

Easyway insures that you escape from the trap permanently by removing your desire to drink.

That 10 percent who live their lives without ever falling for the alcohol trap are subjected to the same brainwashing as everyone else and therefore somewhere in their minds they probably believe that there is some benefit to be enjoyed from drinking. They, like you, are also aware of the misery that alcohol can cause and they're able to rationalize that there is no sense in inflicting that on themselves. They're able to maintain the power of reason because, luckily for them, their reasoning hasn't been affected by addiction.

## EASYWAY DOES NOT REQUIRE WILLPOWER TO RESIST TEMPTATION. IT REMOVES TEMPTATION ALTOGETHER

As long as you retain the desire to drink, you will suffer a feeling of deprivation when you stop. You will have to use willpower to fight this sense of deprivation and you will remain at risk of falling back into the trap for the rest of your life.

Easyway permanently removes the desire to drink so that you do not go through life feeling deprived or having to resist temptation.

If you think that sounds impossible, it's because of the distorted way you see drinking. Nondrinkers have no desire to drink and nor did you until you got hooked. There are also millions of ex-drinkers who once thought they could never get free but have now escaped and have no desire whatsoever to drink again.

Soon you will join them.

## SEE ALCOHOL FOR WHAT IT IS

It's easy for us to recognize the heroin trap. The things we're told about heroin as we're growing up are quite clear: ADDICTION! SLAVERY! POVERTY! MISERY! DEGRADATION! DEATH! But the way alcohol is portrayed is completely different. Happy, beautiful people, having fun or acting cool and sophisticated, showing no signs of strain or anxiety, enjoying all the pleasures that life has to offer. The message is straightforward: "Alcohol makes you happy."

Do you agree with that? I assume you don't, which is why you're reading this book. It's time to blow away these illusions once and for all, so that instead of seeing drinking as a pleasure or support, you will see the true picture, just as you do with heroin. By the time you finish the book your frame of mind will be such that, whenever you think about drinking, instead of feeling deprived because you can no longer drink, you will feel overjoyed because you no longer have to.

If you can look at a heroin addict and see the mistake he's making in thinking the next fix will make everything all right, you're already on the way to solving your own problem. The aim of this book is to help you reverse the brainwashing that's led you into the drinking trap. It will help you to see that drinking does not relieve your misery at all; it's the cause of it. There is no need for you to be miserable. The life of the happy nondrinker awaits you very soon. You have every reason to feel excited.

In choosing to read this book, you have made it clear that you have reached the point in your descent into the alcohol trap where you realize that all is not well. Perhaps you reached that point a long time ago but did not receive the correct instructions to help you escape. Now you want to get out, you want to stop drinking and start living life to the full free from the slavery of alcohol. This book has all the instructions you need to make your escape. It's time to cast off the misery of alcohol addiction and start feeling excited about what you're about to achieve.

My third instruction is:

### *START WITH A FEELING OF ELATION*

From now on, I want you to put the idea that escape will be hard and painful out of your mind. It's a myth. Instead, think about your liberation as a hostage must think about theirs. Think about the light, the space, the freedom, the happiness. Think about your friends and family and how much life you have to share with them. Feel the excitement growing as that freedom draws nearer. Nothing stands in your way now. Just keep following the instructions and your escape is guaranteed.

## SUMMARY

- Your addiction is not a weakness in you, nor something magical in the alcohol. It's a trap.

- The alcohol trap exists in the mind.

- In order to escape permanently we must remove the desire to drink.

- Rejoice! You're on the road to solving your problem.

Chapter 4

# UNDERSTANDING WHY YOU DRINK

*Why are we drawn to alcohol in the first place when we know it poses a threat to our health and happiness?*

Let's begin by examining why we start drinking. Everybody knows the disastrous effects alcohol can have. Nobody is under any illusion that, even in so-called normal drinkers, it debilitates all the bodily functions, in particular the senses and coordination. Listen to the way young people talk about drinking and it appears that these are the very reasons they do it.

"I'm going to get sloshed."

"I want to get legless."

"Let's tie one on."

As children, with relatively little knowledge, we content ourselves with innocent games. As adults, with more knowledge, we deliberately put ourselves in the way of harmful pursuits. Why?

It's a paradox caused by a psychological condition that affects everyone to a certain extent, an emptiness that opens up during our development, starting from birth. I call it "the void" and it affects all of us to different degrees.

It works like this. The shock of birth leaves us desperately seeking security. We reach for our mothers and they protect us. Our neediness and vulnerability continue through childhood, when we're cocooned from the harsh realities of life in a fantasy world of make-believe.

But before long we discover that Santa Claus and fairies do not exist. Worse still, we discover that life isn't forever. Consciousness of our own mortality is frightening. At the same time we're forced from the safety of home, to school and a new set of fears and insecurities. As we enter our teens we look more critically at our parents and it begins to dawn on us that they're not the unshakeable pillars of strength that we had always thought them to be. They have weaknesses, frailties, and fears, just as we do.

The disillusionment leaves a void in our lives that we tend to fill with pop stars, movie stars, TV celebrities or sports heros. We create our own fantasies. We make gods of these people and start to attribute to them qualities far in excess of those that they possess. We try to bask in their reflected glory. Instead of becoming complete, strong, secure, and unique individuals in our own right, we become followers, impressionable fans, leaving ourselves wide open to suggestion.

In the face of all this bewilderment and instability, we begin to look for support, for a little boost now and then. We instinctively look to our role models and, quite naturally, copy the things they appear to be doing for comfort and relaxation: drinking, smoking, gambling, etc.

### CELEBRITY ROLE MODELS

How often do you see celebrities campaigning to raise awareness of the dangers of alcohol? Certainly not as often as you see them endorsing it. Drinking is as much a part of a high society lifestyle as it ever was and among women it has increased dramatically. Whereas, in the early days of showbiz stardom, it was deemed unladylike for a woman to be seen drunk, today the sight of a female celebrity falling out of a nightclub and into a car is a weekly occurrence. Do you think this dissuades impressionable young girls from drinking? On the contrary, it reinforces the myth that drinking is "the thing to do."

Another major influence is our circle of friends. Regardless of what we might think privately about alcohol, when all our friends are drinking we come under immense pressure to join in. Alcohol, after all, is perceived as the sociable drug, the drug we take in groups so we can all get drunk together. Anyone who stands aside from that accepted norm is seen as a party pooper.

It's fair to say that among adults, drinking is considered normal behavior and those who don't drink are regarded as the exception. In this respect alcohol is unlike any other drug. So not only do we have the influence of our role models encouraging us to drink, we also have the pressure of our peer group. We want to fit in, so we continue to drink, and all the facts we know about the harmful effects of alcohol get buried at the back of our minds.

In fact, because of peer pressure, our knowledge of the harm alcohol causes can actually become a reason to drink. As young adults we want to prove that we can handle danger because we perceive that as something adults do.

When we're children, our parents protect us from danger by putting themselves in the way. They make our lives easier by bearing the brunt of life's hardships. Therefore, as we approach adulthood ourselves, we take on the behaviors that we perceive to be adult. Handling danger is seen as a grown-up thing to do, so much so that grown-ups show off by demonstrating just how much danger they can handle.

No wonder we copy that behavior when we first start drinking together in groups. It's a case of no one wanting to be the first to blink.

## THE HIDDEN MESSAGE

There is another way in which the negative messages we're given about drinking and other harmful activities can actually influence us in favor of them. Why is it not enough for us to know that alcohol can cause huge damage? Why do we continue to drink as if it is the greatest thing on Earth?

The answer lies in the way we're brainwashed from birth. During our teenage years, we discover that some of the things we've been warned against are actually pleasurable. This sows a seed in our minds: We suspect that this might be the case with everything we've been warned against. Then we see people we admire enjoying those very things and our suspicions are confirmed.

Rather than take the warnings at face value, we look for a hidden message: "If people are doing it in spite of all the dangers I've been warned about, there must be something great about it."

The simple truth, which we're never told, is that all those influences—the celebrities, the friends, our parents—are drinking because they too have been brainwashed and now they're in the trap.

## THE MONSTERS WITHIN

When I first devised my method I focused exclusively on smoking, but I always knew that it could be applied to alcoholism and other addictions. Although the drug may vary, the principle remains the same.

The addict is deluded into believing the drug provides a genuine pleasure or support, when, in fact, it does the opposite.

As alcohol leaves the body, the withdrawal creates a feeling of unease and emptiness, like a niggling itch. I call this feeling the Little Monster. The Little Monster is created by consuming alcohol. It feeds on alcohol and when you don't give it what it wants, it begins to complain. The feeling is barely perceptible, and the real problem is that it creates another monster.

This second monster is not physical but psychological. I call it the Big Monster and it's created by a combination of the Little Monster and the brainwashing that drinking provides a genuine pleasure or support.

The Big Monster interprets the Little Monster's complaints as "I need or want a drink," and so you end up trying to satisfy the craving by doing the very thing that caused the craving in the first place.

When you consume alcohol it temporarily quietens the Little Monster, creating the illusion that the drink has made you relaxed and happy. In fact, all it has done is taken you from feeling slightly uptight and restless to feeling OK. Before you created the Little Monster you were OK anyway, you didn't need alcohol. Now you will need it again and again just to get you back to a level where you feel OK.

In fact you never quite get back to where you were before you started. The body builds up a tolerance to all addictive drugs, so you never completely relieve the withdrawal even while you are drinking, and so the tendency is to increase your intake. The longer you go on trying to satisfy the Little Monster with alcohol, the lower your wellbeing sinks and the more dependent you feel on the drug.

Drinking never makes you feel fulfilled.

## HOW ALCOHOL WORKS

Alcohol is an anesthetic, and an anesthetic is a drug that kills feelings and sensations. Most people would agree that alcohol can temporarily dull unpleasant feelings. If that is so, how can it possibly enhance pleasant feelings? If it dulls the negative feelings resulting from unpleasant experiences, surely it must also dull the positive feelings resulting from pleasant experiences.

But drinkers will believe anything. We somehow convince ourselves alcohol is some kind of smart bomb: that it wipes out trouble and woe but miraculously leaves pleasant experiences intact—or even enhances them! It cannot possibly work like that. Alcohol deadens the brain. If you consume it to try to reduce your awareness of your cares and worries, there's going to be collateral damage: It will reduce your appreciation of genuine pleasures as well.

Wouldn't you prefer to be fully present for every human experience?

WHY NOT SHOW UP FOR THE ONE LIFE YOU HAVE

## WHY WOULD YOU WANT TO BE "OUT OF IT"?

What's so great about being drunk, or "out of it," as the expression goes? In fact, the terms we use for drunkenness are very revealing. Many are references to bodily functions: for example "bladdered," along with others I could mention; or they refer to the fact that alcohol impairs every one of your faculties: "blind drunk," "legless," and "paralytic;" or the images are of violence, destruction and death: "bombed," "hammered," "blitzed," "slaughtered," "smashed," "trashed," "mashed," "annihilated," "wrecked," and most telling of all, "wasted."

My medical dictionary uses slightly different language. It defines the effects of alcohol as: "deterioration of intellectual and motor functions; lengthening of reaction time; dulling of higher mental processes; impairment of judgment, attention, self-discipline, coordinating skills and visual acuity; and decreasing sensitivity to sensory stimuli."

I came across this medical definition of the symptoms of alcohol intoxication about the time my cat died. She took a while to go, and it struck me the definition could equally apply to the symptoms of dying: She seemed confused and her reactions became slow; we took her for a final walk in the garden and her legs buckled under her; her senses were obviously going—her eyes started to glaze over. The most important point is she was obviously not enjoying herself—it was clearly quite scary for her.

## NOT SO SPECIAL EFFECTS

We've all been programmed to believe that alcohol is wonderful, but imagine what its effects would be like for someone who has never heard of it; who has never been brainwashed or warned about those effects, who hasn't built up a tolerance to them, and has no physical withdrawal or mental craving to try to relieve. Imagine they were tricked into consuming a large amount, and suddenly found themselves unable to think, move, see, or talk properly!

Do you think it would be relaxing?

Do you think it would be pleasant in any way?

No. What do you think it would be like for such a person suddenly to find themselves extremely inebriated?

But perhaps you feel nondrinkers are just goody-goodies

who wouldn't know a good time if it slapped them in the face. That's an opinion shared by many drinkers—at least while they're still drunk.

Is that how you feel when you're sober and someone else is smashed?

When you see a drunken lout reeling around in the street, do they look like they're enjoying themselves?

When some drunk in the street is dribbling down their shirt, do you think: "I wish I was drunk right now!?"

When do you think you're more likely to see inebriation for what it really is: when your judgment has been impaired by a drug, or when you're on the outside looking in?

I'm sure most of us have had this experience at some point in our lives: You're enjoying a relaxing night in and your friends phone you from some bar, drunkenly urging you to join them. Do you want to?

OK, your friends probably think they're having a better time than you. But what would they know? They're out of it!

## DRUNKENNESS IS NO FUN

Of all the drinks you have in a session, with which is there the greatest perception of pleasure? Which is the one that really gives you that "Aaaahh!" feeling: the tenth drink, the third drink, the sixteenth drink, the fifth, the first?

Isn't it the first? And which drink is the one with which you are the least inebriated? Again: the first. That's the one where you hardly even notice the inebriation.

So if the greatest feeling of pleasure is when you are least inebriated, doesn't that imply that it's not the inebriation that creates the feeling of pleasure?

With which drink of the evening is there the least perception of pleasure?

Isn't it the last? Isn't that the drink where there's little if any pleasure? In fact it can be decidedly unpleasant, when your head is spinning or you're throwing up in the gutter. And with which drink of the evening are you most inebriated? Clearly the last. So the greatest perception of pleasure is when you're least inebriated, and there's little if any perception of pleasure when you are at your most inebriated. In fact when you are at your most inebriated, it can be very unpleasant.

So, it's not the inebriation that you're enjoying.

If it were, it would be the other way around: There'd be little if any sense of pleasure with the first drink, and a great sense of pleasure with the last.

If you think the second or third drink is in fact the most pleasurable, that's because you've developed such a high tolerance that you need more than one drink to have any real effect on the Little Monster—in much the same way that a chain-smoker needs to wolf down several cigarettes in the morning to feel any relief. Remember also that it takes around seven minutes for alcohol to reach the brain so that it's perhaps not until your second or third drink that the alcohol from your first reaches your brain and suppresses your withdrawal.

We're confusing two completely separate things. We think

the so-called pleasure and the inebriation are one and the same. They aren't. We think it's the inebriation that gives the sense of pleasure. It isn't. We're mistaking the mere relief of our craving for a pleasurable effect of the drug. We experience that mild inebriation at the same time as the partial relief of the physical withdrawal, and shortly after the relief of the mental craving. So, it's not surprising that the inebriation seems pleasant by association with the relief. We confuse the relief of withdrawal with the inebriation. We think the inebriation and the feeling of pleasure are one and the same thing. They aren't.

## ALCOHOL PROVIDES NO GENUINE PLEASURE

There is nothing genuinely pleasant about inebriation. It may seem pleasant but only because you experience it at exactly the same time as the withdrawal relief.

Most drinkers would claim the sense of pleasure comes from the effect of the drug—from the inebriation. They would claim, in fact, that the sense of pleasure and the inebriation are one and the same thing. Let me prove to you they are two completely different things.

You can feel one without the other. I'm sure you'll agree you can feel inebriated without any sense of pleasure: Your first ever experience of alcohol, for example, and presumably many occasions since. When you're throwing up in the gutter, there's not much pleasure then, is there?

Or let's say you're hammered and you start arguing with your partner—well that's not exactly pleasurable, is it?

So you can be inebriated without any sense of pleasure.

You can also experience the perception of the pleasure of inebriation without being inebriated. In fact you can experience it without having consumed alcohol at all. There have been numerous clever experiments with placebos that demonstrate people will experience the illusion of the pleasure of inebriation from a soft drink they believe to be hard but will not experience it from a hard drink they believe to be soft. Such is the power of the Big Monster.

## WHY WE CONTINUE TO DRINK

We start drinking out of curiosity, peer pressure, or because we believe it must be enjoyable. We're not sure what that pleasure is, but we don't want to miss out, so we try a drink. Most people remember that their first drink tasted foul. If we had that drink without any of the brainwashing that came before it, we would spit it out and never go near it again. But we don't, we persevere. Against everything our instincts are telling us, we continue to drink this foul poison until we're no longer sensitive to the taste. The effect is even more unpleasant as we feel dizzy and the room starts to move and we get a headache and become dehydrated.

It's an extraordinary process, yet 90 percent of adults go through it. If, as I say, we perceive no genuine pleasure in those first drinks, why do we continue to do it? Why is that first experience not enough to put us off completely?

As children we perceive adults to be resilient and strong-willed. They don't give up easily. If they think something's worth fighting for, they'll fight for it. If we're to be perceived as adults, we need to follow suit. "Acquiring a taste" for alcohol may be a revolting ordeal, but we're not about to give in at the first hurdle. We shall overcome! We're convinced that there must be some amazing pleasure to be had from drinking because we see it throughout society. If we didn't experience it the first time, well, we'll just have to try harder, won't we?

So we drink again and we drink more. We've wandered into the trap.

## THE REASON YOU CONTINUE TO DRINK IS THAT YOU'RE CHASING AN IMPOSSIBLE GOAL

I call that goal fulfillment. To begin with, you believe there is some wonderful pleasure to be had from drinking and until you experience that pleasure you feel unfulfilled. Over time, however, drinking does seem to become pleasurable, but by this stage you're in the trap. The only reasons it seems pleasurable are because you have built up a tolerance to the foul taste and have also developed an alcohol addiction, which seems to be relieved by each drink. However, as with all addictive drugs, the body builds up a tolerance not only to the taste but also to the drug itself. This means that you never completely relieve the withdrawal, even while you are drinking, and therefore you remain constantly dissatisfied and unfulfilled.

The tendency is to increase your consumption to try to fill the void, but of course this in turn increases your tolerance. It's a vicious circle. You drink to try to relieve the craving for alcohol caused by your addiction.

Nondrinkers do not have this craving, so, in fact, you drink to feel how a nondrinker feels all the time. The only way you can break the addiction and remove the craving is not to drink. That's why you will never feel fulfilled as long as you keep drinking.

Drinkers believe the only way to relieve their craving for alcohol is to consume the stuff.

In other words, they're deluded into thinking that more alcohol will leave them fulfilled. But what happens when they get their hands on a drink? Do they drink it and stop? Or do they keep on drinking? Remember:

### THE ONLY WAY YOU CAN FEEL LIKE A NONDRINKER IS NOT TO DRINK

Ask a drinker about the feelings that drive them to drink and the answers are very similar to those given by a smoker:

• Boredom—"It's something to do."

• Sadness—"It helps me forget that I'm alone."

• Stress—"It helps me to switch off and forget about my worries."

• Routine—"It's just what I do when the kids have gone

**to bed."**

**• Reward—"It's my treat after a long day."**

In none of these cases does happiness come into it. Sure, we mark happy occasions with a celebratory drink, but that's nothing more than a custom. Our happiness on these occasions doesn't create a need or desire for that drink. In fact, it's when we're happiest that our desire for a drink is lowest. Next time you're at a wedding, make a note of all the unfinished glasses of champagne left on the tables when the dancing begins.

My great pleasure in life is golf. If I could, I would play golf every day. I wouldn't wait until I felt bored, or sad, or stressed. I would break my routine for a game of golf. And I don't feel I have to earn the right to play. I actively pursue it because it gives me pleasure and I know the exercise is good for me.

Addicts often talk about their "drug" in terms of a "reward." But why would anyone "reward" themselves with something that damages their health and wealth, turns them into a different and less likeable person, and destroys their wellbeing?

Addicts aren't stupid; they know the pitfalls. And they know deep down that their drug is not a reward, it's destroying their life. So why do they kid themselves otherwise?

## Because they're caught in an ingenious trap

## THE ILLUSION OF PLEASURE

That first foul-tasting drink is all it takes to trigger a cycle of destruction that can lead to chronic alcoholism. It doesn't matter who you are, how much you earn, where you live or what you do, everyone is vulnerable to the alcohol trap.

Later in the book I will explain why some people become alcoholics and others don't, but at this stage all that matters is that you accept that it has nothing to do with the genetic makeup or personality of the drinker.

Alcohol is a highly addictive drug. As it passes out of your system it leaves an empty, insecure feeling, not dissimilar to hunger. You interpret this feeling as "I want a drink", and think the only way to satisfy it is to have one.

When you have a drink, the empty, insecure feeling is relieved, giving the impression of a little boost. You mistake this boost for pleasure and so it's ingrained in your mind that alcohol gives you pleasure.

But what you're feeling is not genuine pleasure, merely relief from alcohol withdrawal which nondrinkers do not suffer from anyway. You could get the same "satisfaction" by wearing tight shoes all day, just for the "pleasure" of taking them off.

As you increase your intake, the alcohol cravings become more pronounced and, therefore, the illusion of pleasure when you relieve them increases. The more you drink, the more you think it's giving you pleasure. In fact, all it's doing is relieving the discomfort of craving the drug. Nondrinkers don't have that discomfort in the first place.

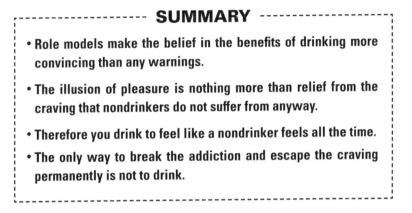

## SUMMARY

- Role models make the belief in the benefits of drinking more convincing than any warnings.

- The illusion of pleasure is nothing more than relief from the craving that nondrinkers do not suffer from anyway.

- Therefore you drink to feel like a nondrinker feels all the time.

- The only way to break the addiction and escape the craving permanently is not to drink.

Chapter 5

# THE TRAP

*All addicts are caught up in an extremely ingenious trap. Whatever the addiction, the trap works in the same subtle and insidious way.*

So, if the craving for a drink is caused by the alcohol from the last drink leaving your system, it should follow that if you can go long enough for all the alcohol to pass out of your body, the cravings should stop and your addiction will be cured. Yet we all know this is not the case. The body is very well equipped for dealing with poisons like alcohol. It takes one hour on average for the liver to metabolize one unit of alcohol and about a week to ten days in most cases for the body to rid itself of all the toxins. Plenty of drinkers have managed to survive a lot longer than ten days without a drink but not managed to rid themselves of the craving. Their only defense against falling back into the trap is willpower, and when their willpower gives out, they start drinking again.

**IN HER OWN WORDS: ANNA**

I managed to stop drinking in April and I was doing really well. Plenty of occasions came and went when I could have had a drink, but I managed to resist and I was feeling really pleased with myself.

Then Christmas came. At the start of December I could feel myself getting into Christmas mode and something inside me started craving a drink. Whether it was the stress of all the preparation or just the time of year being traditionally when I would have drunk a lot, I don't know, but I decided to allow myself a glass of wine.

The next thing I knew I'd drained the whole bottle and was back to square one. I couldn't believe I'd caved in so easily, but if I'm honest, during the seven months I'd been dry, I hadn't gone a single day without wanting a drink. When I finally opened that bottle of wine, it was like welcoming an old lover back into my house— a lover I knew would smash the place up and run off with my money.

The reason we continue to crave a drink even when all traces of alcohol have left our body is that there are two aspects to addiction: a physical aspect and a mental aspect.

The physical addiction goes very quickly once you stop drinking, but if the mental addiction remains you will continue to crave the drug, and as long as you force yourself to go without, you will feel deprived and miserable. Why do you feel deprived? Because you've been deluded into thinking that relief from your misery lies in the drug.

## YOU SEEK SALVATION IN THE VERY THING THAT'S DESTROYING YOU

### GAMBLING ADDICTS

The mental aspect of addiction becomes clear when you look at gambling, one of the most widespread addictions to be gripping the world in the 21st century. Gambling does not involve ingesting a substance, like alcohol, nicotine, or heroin, yet problem gamblers show all the same symptoms as drinkers, smokers, and junkies. It's the illusion of pleasure that hooks them all.

When you're desperate for a drink and finally get your hands on one, how long does it take for the sense of relief to wash over you? Minutes? Hours? No, it's an instant relief, isn't it? You've been dying for that drop of alcohol and finally you have it.

Or have you?

In fact, it's been shown that alcohol takes at least six minutes to reach the brain. So how can that wave of relief be due to the alcohol? It's not.

The craving you have is caused by the belief that alcohol is what you need and so as soon as you think you're getting it, the craving is relieved.

## HOW THE TRAP WORKS

All addicts are caught in the same ingenious trap. When I describe how the trap works for drinkers, you'll see how this is the case. The trap is similar to a pitcher plant, which lures flies into its digestive chamber with the sweet smell of nectar. The plant is shaped like

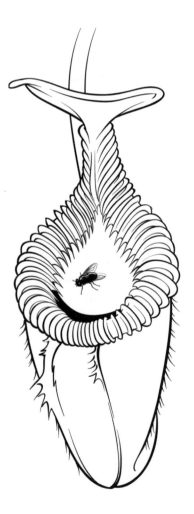

a funnel, the inside of which is coated in a sweet, slippery nectar and at the bottom is a pit containing liquid. The fly lands on the rim and begins to drink. As it does so it feels itself slipping down the funnel towards the pit, in which the drowned bodies of other flies are slowly being digested. But instead of flying away, the fly continues to drink. The nectar tastes good —it seems like the best thing in the world, but it's the very thing that is luring the fly to its death.

Just as the full horror of its predicament doesn't dawn on the fly until it's past the point of no return and it realizes that it can't escape, drinkers don't realize they're stuck in the trap until they're well and truly hooked. They believe that they're in control and drinking because they enjoy it. Only when they try to quit do they realize they're trapped.

We're aware of the arguments against alcohol. We know that it can have a devastating effect on our health and wealth, that it can make us obnoxious, irrational, violent, and impossible to live with. We know that it distorts our judgment and leaves us vulnerable to all manner of abuses. In short, we're armed with enough information to deduce that drinking is something to be avoided.

Yet we also know that millions of people, including most of the adults we know, drink on a regular basis without losing everything they love and possess. And at the same time, the alcoholic drinks industry bombards us with all manner of inducements, from cheap deals on booze in supermarkets to advertisements designed to create the illusion that drinking makes you cool, funny, sophisticated, even intelligent! You only have to watch a drunk spill out of a bar and try to walk home to see that the opposite is true.

The first drink tastes foul. In some cultures a boy becomes a man by having sticks skewered through his skin. We drink alcohol. It may not be quite as painful, but it's not pleasant. Because we see it as a rite of passage into maturity, we persevere until eventually we can down that drink without wanting to throw up.

Now we feel pretty pleased with ourselves. We've achieved that coveted state of being able to "take our drink" and we now relish each opportunity to prove our prowess.

## WE'RE ALREADY LOSING CONTROL

In the early days we're able to con ourselves that we remain in control of when and how much we drink and that there will be no problems. However, as time goes on and the void left after each drink increases as our tolerance builds up, so the illusion of pleasure is magnified each time we relieve it. But it's taking more and more drink to try to relieve the craving and we begin to sense that we're slipping further and further into a bottomless pit. It's an unpleasant, insecure feeling that creates further anxiety and stress.

Just as we reach for the painkillers to numb an aching tooth, we reach for a temporary fix to take away this unpleasant feeling: we drink again. Rather than dealing with the real cause of the problem, we use the temporary fix of our addiction as an anesthetic.

Like any anesthetic, it soon wears off. Now, because the problem has not been addressed, the stress is worse than before. The need for a painkiller is intensified. We drink again, and we drink more in order to feel the effect. The highs become more short-lived, the lows more intense, and the net effect is an increasingly rapid descent towards oblivion, like the fly sliding into the belly of the pitcher plant.

This is how the trap works. It's how any addiction works.

## THE ADDICT SEEKS RELIEF IN THE VERY THING THAT'S CAUSING THE MISERY

**NATURE'S WARNING LIGHT**

The way we try to anesthetize our pain is an example of how easy it is to fool our intellect. Say you have a toothache; you take a painkiller. After a while the pain subsides and you feel better. But has the problem with your tooth gone away? Not at all. The pain has just been suppressed.

But the pain was serving a useful purpose: It was telling your brain and body that there's a problem with your teeth that needs sorting out. By suppressing the pain and dealing with the symptom rather than the cause, you prevent your body from responding to the problem appropriately.

Imagine you're driving a car and the oil light comes on. What do you do? Remove the bulb from the warning indicator? Or pull over and top up the oil? Both actions will stop the oil light from flashing; only one will prevent the engine from seizing up.

## AN INEVITABLE DECLINE

The human body is an incredible machine with a remarkable facility for recovery and adaptation. Feed it poison and it will react violently to eject the poison from your system. That's why drinking makes you vomit. At the same time it will build a defensive tolerance to the poison, so that next time it takes more poison to create the same effect.

I've said we drink in order to feel how a nondrinker feels all the time. In fact, we never quite achieve the fulfillment of a nondrinker. How can we when each drink only partially relieves the withdrawal and our physical and mental health is continuously declining?

## THE ONLY WAY TRULY TO FEEL LIKE A NONDRINKER IS TO STOP DRINKING

We get used to feeling below par—it becomes our new sense of "normal"—but as we continue to crave a drink we drop lower and lower (see diagram opposite). If the nondrinker's "normal" is at 0 on this graph, let's say a drinker in the early stages is at -4 because of the overall decline in physical and mental health. As the craving goes unsatisfied, your wellbeing falls to -10. Now you have a drink, the craving is partially relieved and you experience a boost up to -5. You don't quite get back to -4 because you can never fully relieve the withdrawal from alcohol while you continue to drink.

As the alcohol leaves your system again, the withdrawal increases and your wellbeing level falls. You are experiencing a double low: the physical low of withdrawal and the mental low of craving another drink. When you have a drink, both lows are relieved, increasing the illusion of a boost but still not getting you back up to where you started. Alcohol debilitates you both physically and mentally and as you go through life your wellbeing is constantly declining, so the lows get lower and lower and the highs also decline in proportion.

Each time you drink, you need a bigger boost to get you anywhere near to where you started. But it never puts you back on par. And so you go on, falling by ever-increasing amounts. While each little peak continues to mislead you into believing that drinking is giving you a boost, the reality is that your wellbeing is continuously declining, particularly as it becomes increasingly obvious that you've become a slave to alcohol.

## *THE ADDICTION HAS TAKEN HOLD*

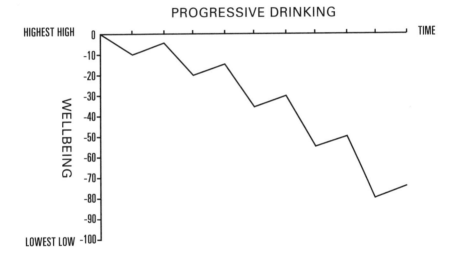

Can you see the connection with the pitcher plant? At what point would you say the fly lost control?

When it started slipping down the inside of the plant?

No, it must have been before that.

When it tried to fly away and found it couldn't?

That was the point at which it realized it had lost control, so it must have happened before that too.

What about when it saw all the other dead insects at the bottom of the plant, or even before that, when it landed on the lip of the plant?

It could have escaped at either point had it wanted to. But it didn't want to. Why? Because it didn't realize it was in a trap.

In fact, the fly was never in control. It was being subtly controlled by the plant from the moment it first caught the aroma of the nectar. The same is true of all drinkers. From the moment we're drawn to that first drink, we're controlled by alcohol.

The good news is that all those points on the graph are recoverable when you quit drinking. Remember, the fact that you've fallen into the trap has nothing to do with your character or personality. Millions of people, who have found themselves in the same trap and been convinced that they will never be able to escape, have gotten free and so will you.

Consider the bad effects of your drinking as the equivalent of the unsightly fat on somebody who is overweight, or as the smoker's cough or the threat of lung cancer. You try to cover them up, you pretend they're not there, you kid yourself that they're under control, you'll deal with them soon, just not yet. But these are ever-increasing, dark shadows looming at the back of your mind and as you slip further and further into the trap, they loom larger and larger, and get darker and darker.

Like the fly, you only realize you're trapped by drinking when you're well and truly hooked. But there is one crucial difference between the pitcher plant and the alcohol trap:

## IT'S NEVER TOO LATE TO ESCAPE FROM THE ALCOHOL TRAP

Unlike the fly, you're not standing on a slippery slope; there is no physical force compelling you to drink more. The trap is entirely in your mind. The fact that you're your own jailer is an ingenious aspect of the trap and fortunately for you, it's also its fatal flaw. You have the power to escape simply by understanding the nature of the trap and following the easy instructions in this book.

## WHAT'S STOPPING YOU FROM FLYING FREE?

When you see the trap in these terms, the solution looks simple: stop drinking and just fly away. But as you know, when you're actually in the trap, nothing looks simple. That's because there are two major illusions corrupting your judgment:

1. The myth that drinking gives you pleasure and/or support.

2. The myth that escape will be hard and painful.

You probably have good memories of certain times when you've drunk heavily: parties, celebrations, weekends away with friends. But where did the real pleasure come from on those occasions? Was it really the drinking that made your day? Or was it the company of your friends, the banter you had between you, the sheer pleasure of being with people you like?

Take away the drinking and the situation would still have been enjoyable. Take away the company and the drinking would have been no fun.

"But if the brain can be deceived into believing that drinking makes us happy, does it matter that it isn't true?"

Yes it does, because while the brain may be deceived, the opposite is true. Moreover, you're risking your health, your job, your relationships, not to mention wasting your money and finding those joyful occasions more and more difficult to come by. There's only so long you can go on burying your head in the sand before these grim realities take a very heavy toll.

As the fly is descending into the pitcher plant, there's a point at which it senses that all is not well and thinks about flying out. For the fly, this point usually comes too late. It's physically stuck. For you there is no physical force preventing your escape and yet, when you sense that you're being consumed by drinking and want to get free, you find you cannot. You know that the only way to free yourself from this misery is to stop drinking and yet the thought of doing so is so daunting that you would rather bury your head in the sand and keep sliding into the trap than face the ordeal of escape. You have fallen for the myth that escape has to be hard and painful.

At any point on our descent into the alcohol trap, we could stop and walk back out, easily and painlessly. And yet, because we have been led to believe otherwise, and may have tried the willpower method which involves feeling deprived and miserable, we are convinced that it will be hard, with the result that we either repeatedly put off making the attempt or we start the attempt feeling we're making a terrible sacrifice. Both have the same result: we remain in the trap.

The reason we believe that escape will be hard and painful is that we have been convinced that drinking gives us some form of pleasure or support and, therefore, stopping would mean making a sacrifice. It's time we unraveled the illusions that have been keeping you in the alcohol trap.

## SUMMARY

- Addicts seek relief in the very thing that's causing the problem.
- The pleasure you feel is not the effect of the drug itself, it's the relief of your craving.
- Your physical and mental wellbeing is constantly eroded when you continue to drink.
- The myth of pleasure and the erroneous belief it is hard to escape keep you trapped.
- It's never too late to fly free and recapture the joy of being a nondrinker.

Chapter 6

# ILLUSIONS

**IN THIS CHAPTER**

•*INSTINCT V INTELLECT*

•*DISTINGUISHING TRUTH FROM MYTH*

•*I LIKE THE TASTE*

*It's widely thought that alcohol provides a genuine pleasure or crutch. I'll explain why this is never actually the case.*

The myth that drinking gives you pleasure or support and the myth that stopping will be hard and painful are the two main illusions that prevent drinkers from quitting and sometimes from even making the attempt. But if I were in your shoes, I would be asking two burning questions right now:

1.  How do I know that they are illusions? Maybe Easyway is just trying to con me that they are to help me to stop.

2.  How could so many people succumb to these illusions, including me?

Let's deal with the second question first. I admit, it seems incredible that the most sophisticated creature on the planet could fall for illusions that cause it such massive harm. After all, are humans not the great survivors? We have devised ways to survive and thrive that have made us more powerful than any other species on Earth.

The vital difference between human beings and wild animals is that animals survive solely by instinct. Humans also use instinct to survive: It tells us when and what to eat, it alerts us to danger, it even helps us to find a suitable mate. But we have another tool, which has enabled us to rule over the animal kingdom: intellect.

Our intellect has given us the capacity to learn and pass on our learning, with the result that we have developed into a highly sophisticated species that is capable of building fantastic structures and machines and also has an appreciation of art, music, romance, spirituality and so on.

Intellect is a wonderful thing, but it can go to your head; for it's our intellect that has also led us astray. Instinct is nature's survival kit, but there are times when it conflicts with our intellect and then we tend to trust the things we've learned over our instincts.

Why? Because instinct often gives us the answer we don't want to hear. An example is the sportsman who needs a painkilling injection in order to play. His instincts are giving the clear signal to rest and allow the injury to recover but his intellect tells him he can numb the pain and play on.

That's the answer he wants to hear because he's desperate to play. So he plays, and the result can be irreversible damage to his body. His instinct was right, yet he chose to side with his intellect.

Look again at the "advances" mankind has made and you'll see that, rather than building on the advantage that nature has given us, we've devoted a remarkable amount of time, effort, and resources to self-destruction.

I don't just mean the ever more sophisticated ways of killing each other in battle, the intellectual choice of self-destruction is also evident in the food we eat. We have become a species of compulsive junk food consumers. How? By allowing our intellect to trick our instincts.

### SUGAR SUGAR

The reason we're so partial to refined sugar and all the candy, cakes, drinks, etc. that contain it, is that it mimics the natural sugar in fruit. Fruit is the food that nature designed us to eat and our taste for the natural sugars in fruit is designed to keep us coming back for more. Refined sugar contains none of the goodness of fruit, yet it tricks our taste buds into thinking it's the same thing. Intellectually we have created a substance that fools our instincts into thinking we're getting something good when, in truth, it's bad.

This ability of our intellect to trick our instincts lies behind most of the harm we do to ourselves as a species. When we make intellectual choices based on misinformation—like eating sugary foods because our taste buds are fooled—our wellbeing begins to suffer. Wild animals do not experience bouts of self-loathing.

Intellect causes misery just as it causes happiness. The choice is ours. So why do we so often take the self-destructive option?

Quite simply because we don't always realize we have an option. Nobody chooses to become a drinker for the rest of their life. There are always people who stand to gain as a result of these destructive human practices, be they arms dealers, drug cartels, the tobacco and alcoholic drinks industries, fast food chains, or gambling firms, and they have become masters at exploiting our intellect to pass on false information.

It's not hard to trick the human mind. We proved that with the table illusion in Chapter 2. Take a look at this jumble of shapes. What does it say to you?

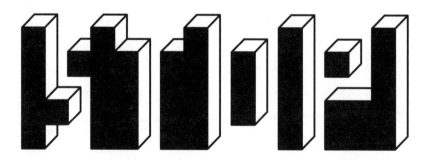

Is there a coherent message in it all? At first it can look like a random line of building blocks. There isn't really a meaningful message there at all, is there?

Now look again. This time, look at the shapes with your eyes half-closed and, by peering through your eyelashes, you can make a word appear. It might help if you move your head back a little (or to the side) and look at it from a distance.

Remember, you're not looking at the black type, you're looking at the white space between the type.

You should see the word STOP. Have you got it now? Obvious, isn't it? In fact, now that you can see it, I defy you to look at the same diagram and not see the word STOP. Now that you can see the pattern in the image, the truth should stay with you forever.

So why wasn't it obvious in the first place? Because we're programmed to look for information in the black type on a white page, and the thought of doing the opposite doesn't cross our minds. This is a graphic example of how easy it is to create confusion between your instinct and your intellect. The way addictions work is to create a false sense of pleasure and reward through the ingenious con trick of withdrawal relief, which your mind comes to mistake for the real thing.

I have explained how so many people (most of the human race, in fact) get brainwashed in this way. Now we can address the first question:

### HOW DO I KNOW THAT EASYWAY IS NOT JUST CONNING ME THAT THEY ARE ILLUSIONS?

When you see through an illusion and recognize the truth, you can never be fooled into seeing the illusion again. You fell into the alcohol trap because you were under the illusion that drinking gave you pleasure and/or support. And yet drinking has not made you happy or secure; it has made you miserable and afraid. The truth is there for all to see and, just like the STOP diagram, once you've seen it, nothing will be able to change your perception.

That's how you can distinguish the truth from the myths. So let's take a closer look at some more of these illusions.

## IT TASTES GREAT

Have you ever tasted neat alcohol? I advise you not to. It's pure poison and half a pint drunk neat is enough to kill you. Yet the alcohol industry has succeeded in convincing most of the world that its product tastes great.

We are so eager to convince ourselves that we drink this stuff for the taste, rather than merely to relieve our craving for alcohol, that we join beer or wine appreciation societies and spend long evenings discussing the relative merits of a cheeky sauterne or a nutty real ale. Nutty is the word!

If you need reminding how alcoholic drinks really taste, then think back to the first time you tried one. Who can honestly say that the first time they tasted beer, or wine, or whiskey or any other alcoholic drink, they thought it tasted delicious? Wasn't it the exact opposite? Wasn't your immediate instinct to spit it out and never let it near your lips again?

All alcoholic drinks taste repulsive the first time we try them, so why don't we drop the very idea there and then and never go near alcohol again? Because in just about every case there is a more experienced drinker with us, telling us, "Oh, that's normal. No one likes it the first time. It's an acquired taste. Keep drinking."

In other words, we're led to believe that this is something worth pursuing; that after a while we will acquire the taste for booze and then a door will open on to a whole new world of pleasures. As you now know, this last point could not be further from the truth, but don't feel bad towards the person who told you that. They were told it themselves once, and their experience will have led them to believe it's true. They will have persevered until they stopped finding the taste repulsive and in doing so they will have walked into the alcohol trap, and so they now believe that alcohol gives them some form of pleasure or support.

The reason we don't abstain from drinking after the very first taste is because we want to like it. We feel it's important to like it —that we'll be missing out on something in life if we don't. If you knew then what you know now, would you have persevered in order to "acquire the taste?" The truth is:

## YOU DON'T ACQUIRE THE TASTE FOR ALCOHOL AT ALL; YOU ACQUIRE THE LACK OF TASTE NECESSARY TO STAND IT

Have you ever considered what your tastebuds are designed to do? These days, because everything we eat and drink is packaged up and presented to us without us having to go out and gather it, we tend to regard our taste buds as merely the means for appreciating all the lovely things we consume. But they're designed for a much more important purpose than that.

In the days before our food came to us wrapped up and labeled, we had to go out and find it, and that meant trying foods until we found the ones that were good for us. How did we tell the difference? We tasted and smelled. If we found a fruit that was unripe, it tasted bitter and we spat it out. If it was overripe, it smelled bad and we wouldn't touch it.

When you took that first sip of alcohol, the same reaction took place. Your taste buds detected poison and your instincts rejected it. But in persevering with this foul taste, you overrode your natural warning mechanism and began to build up a tolerance to the poison.

Society calls this "acquiring the taste"—in fact, you've acquired a lack of taste.

When it comes to drinking, our taste buds are designed to find the best thing we can to quench our thirst. Imagine you'd spent two days walking across the desert and I found you gasping with thirst. I offered you a glass of water and a glass of wine. Which would you reach for?

When people say they love a cold, thirst-quenching beer, they forget that beer is 95 percent water. Their thirst would be better quenched by a glass of pure water, but the effect of the cold beer for the drinker is more powerful, because it relieves the craving for alcohol at the same time.

Of course, alcohol is a diuretic, which means it dehydrates you. Therefore, the alcohol doesn't quench your thirst at all; it works against the thirst-quenching effects of the water and leaves you wanting more.

That's why people manage to put away pint after pint of beer in one evening. They couldn't do that with water; their thirst would be quickly satisfied.

If there is a pleasant taste to any alcoholic drink, it comes not from the alcohol but from other ingredients. We seldom drink spirits neat and usually mix them with fruit: vodka and orange, gin and lime, brandy, and cola, etc.

As tolerance to the poison builds up, you start to focus on these flavors and, of course, these are flavors we were designed to enjoy because they're the flavors of fruit. Fruit gives us vital vitamins and water too. It's the ideal food for human beings, and so it's not surprising that the tastes we enjoy most are fruit flavors.

Why, then, don't soft drinks give us the same satisfaction?

The fact is they do; it just depends on the situation. Go back to the desert analogy: In such circumstances a soft drink would be much more satisfying than an alcoholic one.

The times when we might not find soft drinks satisfying are when we've been programmed to expect alcohol: in a bar, out to dinner, at a party.

The conclusion is obvious: it's our craving for alcohol that makes us drink booze on these occasions. It has nothing to do with the taste.

I like a curry. I'm particularly fond of chicken bhuna. I find it impossible to walk past an Indian restaurant without salivating. But if someone told me I could never have a chicken bhuna again, I would feel slightly deprived, but I wouldn't let it get me down. I certainly wouldn't put my health and happiness at risk for one. Can you honestly say that you go through all the misery that alcohol causes you because you like the taste?

## SUMMARY

- The alcoholic drinks industry exploits us by feeding us false information about drinking.

- Once you see the truth from the myth, you can never be fooled by the myth again.

- You don't acquire a taste for alcohol, you acquire a lack of taste.

- You don't drink alcohol for the taste, you drink it to get the drug.

Chapter 7

# I WANT A DRINK

**IN THIS CHAPTER**
•*SOCIAL OCCASIONS* •*IMPAIRED JUDGEMENT*
•*IT RELAXES ME* •*IT'S JUST A HABIT*
•*IT'S THE WAY I'M MADE* •*CONTRADICTIONS*

*One of the most powerful illusions among drinkers is that they cannot enjoy or cope with life without alcohol.*

At the end of the last chapter I gave three examples of occasions when a soft drink is often considered unsatisfactory: in a bar, out to dinner, at a party. This leads us to the most common excuse for drinking: that it helps to make social occasions more enjoyable.

We often go into social occasions with a lack of confidence. Will I know anyone there? Will they find me interesting? Will I meet anyone I like? One of the key aspects that makes social occasions fun is surely that we don't know exactly what's going to happen. Who wants a party to be predictable?

Nevertheless, these questions raise fears within us and so we reach for our little crutch to quell those fears. We have been brainwashed into believing that alcohol gives us courage.

The term "Dutch courage" originates from the days when English troops were given Dutch gin to calm their nerves before going into battle. There's an important distinction here: it may well have calmed their nerves by knocking out those particular emotions, but it didn't give them anything, least of all courage.

Courage is acting in spite of fear. A fireman who runs into a burning building to rescue a baby is not fearless—he knows only too well the danger he's in and any fully conscious human who is in danger will feel fear. Yet he sets the fear for his own life aside to save the life of the baby. That is true courage.

Just as taste buds have a very valuable purpose, so does fear. It's the emotion that alerts us to danger, by triggering the "fight or flight" response. If we block out that response with alcohol, we're leaving ourselves vulnerable.

### CHECK YOUR INSTRUMENTS

Imagine a pilot flying over a mountain range in cloud. He knows he needs to fly at a certain altitude to avoid the peaks, and he gauges his altitude by looking at his altimeter. If he looks at the altimeter and sees he's flying too low, he may feel a momentary surge of panic but he will respond quickly and pull the plane up to a safe height. The altimeter is his constant gauge of danger from the mountains and as long as it keeps working and he keeps responding to it, he will remain safe.

But suppose the altimeter malfunctions. Its little warning light that flashes when the plane drops too low stops working. The pilot thinks everything's fine but

> really he's hurtling towards the mountains. Suddenly a peak looms out of the cloud and he realizes the danger he's in.

It's a mistake to regard fear as debilitating. As this example shows, it's the absence of fear that is debilitating. There is nothing genuinely frightening about a social occasion, but there are dangers associated with them, such as getting home in one piece and, for women in particular, making sure you don't leave yourself vulnerable to ill-intentioned men.

When we're in real danger, we need all our faculties to be fully functional: the ability to run, to shout, to fight, to think. Fear triggers all these responses. Block out fear with alcohol and you're effectively burying your head in the sand. The effect is twofold: You not only fail to identify danger when it arises, you also lack the ability to respond effectively.

Here's a reminder of a few expressions we use for being drunk:

Blind drunk

Legless

Paralytic

Wasted

Is it really necessary to debilitate all your bodily functions in order to enjoy social occasions?

In the longer term, drinking to give yourself courage has a further ill effect. If you have fears, drinking may dull them but it won't make them go away. On the contrary, as you become less capable of tackling whatever it is that is frightening you, the fear increases. Imagine a girl who finds herself in the home of a strange man she's met in a bar. She's drunk, he seemed attractive, she trusted him. Now she's getting cold feet. He seems a bit odd and she realizes she's alone in his apartment, completely at his mercy. She's struggling to stand up, let alone fight or run. How frightened do you think she feels?

I'm not trying to scare you with horror stories. I'm just trying to show how fear gives us the ability to protect ourselves and the ability to protect ourselves alleviates fear. Interfere with this and both your vulnerability and your fear will increase. You create a vicious circle: The more you turn to alcohol to quell your fear, the more your fear increases, so the more you turn to alcohol. This is how the alcohol trap works. It's like a pitcher plant, dragging you further and further down, while you think that it's giving you support.

## IMPAIRING YOUR INHIBITIONS

Shyness is not an unattractive trait. Who would you rather spend time in conversation with, someone who doesn't talk much but listens, or someone who talks too much and shows no interest in what you have to say?

Social occasions may make shy people feel vulnerable, but any sense of inadequacy is only in their own mind. Brash, talkative, and drunk people may hog the limelight and thus create the superficial impression that they're more entertaining than everyone else. In fact, most people are secretly wishing they would shut up and give someone else a chance.

But because these motormouths seem so self-assured, we want a bit of what they have and so we turn to alcohol. But alcohol doesn't make us more interesting; it just removes our ability to tell when we're being dull.

What is shyness? Is it not a form of fear: the fear of making a fool of oneself? Just as fear protects us from danger, so shyness protects us from humiliation. Of course, shy people tend to have a heightened sense of fear before social occasions, but that's no different from an actor getting nervous before going on stage. Once you're in the situation, you deal with it and your confidence grows. Try to drown your shyness with booze and you increase the likelihood of making a fool of yourself.

Disabling your inhibitions with alcohol is tantamount to removing the bulb from your oil warning light. The threat doesn't go away, only your awareness of it disappears.

Making a fool of yourself is one thing—and with drunks it's a very common thing—but there are other inhibitions that, when knocked out, can lead to far more serious consequences. I refer back to the vulnerable girl who goes home with a strange man at the end of the evening. Sober, she would be acutely aware of the risks involved in such an action. Drunk, her reading of the situation is impaired and she puts herself in danger.

You could say that good manners are a form of inhibition, whereby we control our thoughts about someone in order not to hurt their feelings or cause antagonism. Drunks often become rude and abusive.

Why? Because the sense that inhibits rudeness is blocked

out. They also become aggressive and accuse people of being rude to them.

We have many social skills designed to help maintain a civilized society: politeness, tolerance, tact, diplomacy, the ability to listen, the ability to show an interest in others, the ability to pacify. Alcohol impairs all these skills and the results are what we regard as stereotypical drunken behavior:

Insensitivity

Long-windedness

Rudeness

Impatience

Abusiveness

Boorishness

Aggression

Violence

In the case of the latter, the inability to know when to stop can have frightening, even deadly consequences. It's very rare for two sober people to come to blows. In most cases, there's a lot of talk and posturing as both parties go through the primitive ritual of trying to face their opponent down. Neither one wants to hit or be hit and in most cases they will back down before it comes to that.

Add alcohol to the mix, however, and the sense that inhibits violence is blocked out. The primitive instincts that enable us to assess the situation and weigh up our chances of emerging unscathed—or, indeed, inflicting grievous harm – stop working. A small man will take on a big man, believing he can win. And despite being soundly beaten, he will not concede. On the flip side, the fighter who has his opponent beaten does not know when to stop and keeps pummeling until someone drags him off. What if there is no one to drag him off?

Perhaps you think I'm painting an unbalanced picture. Sure, most social occasions pass off without anyone getting hospitalized or killed in a drunken fight, but I'm citing these extreme examples —and they're by no means uncommon—to illustrate the point that applies when going into any social occasion:

## ALCOHOL DOESN'T GIVE YOU ANY POWERS; IT TAKES YOUR POWERS AWAY

No doubt you will have experienced numerous happy social occasions where a lot of drink has been consumed, and you will assume that it was the drink that oiled the wheels. But think about it: Who were you with and what were you doing? Isn't it the case that those occasions were really enjoyable because of the company and the occasion? A wedding, a birthday, a baseball game, a Christmas party.

The belief that alcohol is necessary to have a good time leads many people to spoil the occasion and have a bad one. Once you've freed yourself from alcohol and learned once again to trust in your ability to relate to other people and have fun, just as we do as children, you will go into all social occasions with greater confidence and come out having had more enjoyment than ever.

## *IT RELAXES ME*

It's a classic scenario, acted out time and time again on TV and in the movies, as well as in real life. A person comes home after a long, hard day, kicks off their shoes, flops into an armchair, and says, "I could murder a drink." They're stressed, their nerves are frayed, and they believe that alcohol will help them unwind. In fact, the opposite is true.

Nerves and stress, like fear, serve an important purpose. They alert us to problems. Sometimes the problem is simply that we're overdoing it. If we don't heed the warning signs and do something about it, we run the risk of grinding to a halt.

It's the oil warning light syndrome again. Stress and nerves are a sign that we need to do something to take care of ourselves. If we remove that warning sign with alcohol, the problem doesn't go away, it gets worse. And so the stress increases.

In fact, the effect is twofold because alcohol is also a major cause of stress. As it leaves your system it creates a restless, insecure feeling, which you interpret as "I want a drink." Until you satisfy that feeling, you will feel stressed and nervous.

"Ah!" you might say. "But if alcohol gives the impression of relieving stress, what does it matter if it doesn't actually do so?"

Because it not only causes stress but also has numerous other undesirable effects.

The feeling of relaxation you experience is the partial relief of the uncomfortable feeling of withdrawing from alcohol brought about by the previous drink.

## IT'S AS ILLOGICAL AS WEARING TIGHT SHOES, JUST TO GET THE RELIEF OF TAKING THEM OFF

While you go on believing it relieves stress, you're failing to address the real cause of your stress and the real damage to your health is getting worse. It's like responding to the oil warning light by topping up with sand. The light might go out but the engine is doomed!

Remember, as alcohol leaves your body you start to feel uptight. If you have a drink, you do feel more relaxed. That is not an illusion. But all you're trying to do is relieve the withdrawal caused by the Little Monster, which nondrinkers do not suffer anyway. In fact, the more you drink, the more stressed you become.

## ALCOHOL PREVENTS YOU FROM UNWINDING

Kick off your shoes, change your clothes, take a shower, eat something, flop in your armchair… all these actions will help to relieve the discomforts of a long, hard day. Alcohol will not.

## IT'S JUST A HABIT

The words habit and addiction are often used synonymously these days. People talk about a "drug habit." But there is a clear distinction between them and it's absolutely essential that you understand what it is, otherwise you won't fully grasp either the nature of the victim or of the trap, and you will always be vulnerable.

With habits, you're in control. They might be unpleasant habits, but you do them only because you want to. Habits are easy to break provided you want to break them. We drive on the left in the U.K. but have no difficulty switching to the right when abroad. The important thing is the underlying reason why certain behavior becomes habitual. That reason might be beneficial. If so, why break the habit? It's unlikely anyone would deliberately get into the habit of repeating behavior that provided them with no benefit, unless, of course, they were deluded into believing that an evil was beneficial: as in the case of alcohol addiction.

Drinkers believe that they choose to drink because it gives them some kind of pleasure or support, but if, at any time, they were to take their head out of the sand and list all the advantages and disadvantages of drinking alcohol, the conclusion would be, "You're a fool. Stop doing it!" This is why all drinkers and all other addicts instinctively feel stupid.

In fact, they're not stupid. There is a powerful force that more than balances the scales, and that force is called addiction. But while you believe it's just habit that compels you to drink, what you're really saying is, "I don't understand why I drink. I don't believe that I get any genuine pleasure from it. It's just a habit I've gotten into and, providing I can survive long enough without a drink, time will solve the problem and my craving will eventually go."

But you would be kidding yourself.

The only way truly to escape from the alcohol trap is to understand how the trap works and how you fell into it in the first place. Only then will you be free from the temptation to fall back in. I don't mean you will resist the temptation, I mean there will be no temptation. You will have no need or desire to drink.

## IT'S THE WAY I'M MADE

Closely tied to the habit illusion is the belief that your drink problem is a symptom of your personality. Either you put your failed attempts to quit down to a weakness in your temperament —a lack of willpower—or to a predisposition to drink, over which you have no control—an addictive personality.

Either excuse is a cop-out. What you're effectively saying is, "I'm powerless to stop drinking and, therefore, I have no choice but to carry on doing it."

The problem is that the bulk of information we receive about addictions such as drinking, smoking, and gambling is that you do need willpower to quit and that there is such a thing as an addictive personality. The fact that this misinformation is disseminated by reputable organizations, which, I have no doubt, act with purely good intentions, only adds to its potency. Why would an organization that genuinely wants to help people stop drinking disseminate misinformation that serves to imprison them more deeply in the trap? The simple answer is because they too have been brainwashed.

Remember the STOP diagram. Once you look at it in a different way and see the true message, you can never be fooled by the illusion again. That's why I asked you to keep an open mind and follow the instructions: because the truth is often the complete opposite of what we assume it to be.

The belief that your alcohol problem is down to a flaw in your personality is a form of denial. Rather than accepting that you have an addiction and taking the necessary steps to overcome it you can say, "I have no choice but to carry on doing it." But why would any problem drinker want to say that? Why would anyone who is suffering the misery and slavery of alcohol addiction make an excuse that took away their option to walk free?

The answer is the fear that they can't cope without alcohol; the fear that they can't enjoy social occasions or handle stress without alcohol; the fear that they have to go through some terrible trauma to get free; and the fear that even if they do manage to stop, they will have to spend the rest of their life resisting the craving.

## THE FACT IS, ALL THESE FEARS ARE CAUSED BY ALCOHOL AND THEY ARE ALL ILLUSIONS. NONDRINKERS DO NOT SUFFER ANY OF THESE FEARS. YOU DRINK BECAUSE YOU ARE ADDICTED TO ALCOHOL

But drinkers, like all addicts, lie. They lie to themselves and to others. The reason they lie is to perpetuate the illusions that enable them to kid themselves that they're in control. But if the alternative is honesty and freedom, why on Earth do they opt for lies and imprisonment?

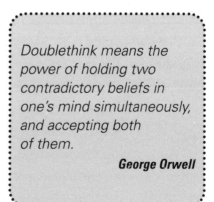

*Doublethink means the power of holding two contradictory beliefs in one's mind simultaneously, and accepting both of them.*

**George Orwell**

The answer can be encapsulated in the word which lies at the root of all addictions:

*FEAR*

---

### SUMMARY

- Alcohol impairs your ability to judge situations.
- Alcohol impairs your social skills.
- Alcohol causes stress and fear.
- Shyness and inhibition serve a useful purpose. So do nerves and stress.

---

Chapter 8

# FEAR

*Drinkers are caught in a tug-of-war of fear which makes them dread even making the attempt to quit.*

Drinkers make excuses for continuing to drink because they're afraid of trying to quit. They believe drinking provides them with a genuine pleasure or support and fear life without it. At the same time, they're aware of the harm they're inflicting on themselves and their loved ones and they're afraid of where it might end up.

This tug-of-war of fear is typical of addiction. You hear it in the things addicts say:

"I know it's destroying my life but it's my last little crutch."

"I'm afraid of losing my family but I can't imagine life without booze."

Fear is both an instinctive and an intellectual response. As discussed in the last chapter, instinct drives us to fight or flight, alerting us to danger and making us wary in potentially dangerous situations. As such it's vital to our survival. But the things that make us fearful can be real or imaginary. Our intellect has enabled us to learn about potential dangers and how to avoid them, so much so that we can be fearful of dangers of which there is no evidence.

The fears associated with losing our job, for example, are intellectual. We have learned about the possible consequences of finding ourselves unemployed—e.g. having no money, being forced to sell our possessions, sacrificing the pleasures and comforts that we enjoy now—and so we do everything in our power to safeguard our job and make ourselves indispensible, even when there is no immediate threat of losing it.

In this instance our intellect is very helpful. But what if your fears are based on false information? Say, for example, you read in a magazine that fruit causes cancer. You would probably avoid eating fruit. You would also worry about the damage already done by all the fruit you've eaten in your life.

I have yet to hear anyone claim that fruit causes cancer, but it's typical of the sort of scare stories with which we're bombarded on a regular basis. Some of them are based on sound evidence, others are absurd. As consumers, it's impossible for us to know what to believe and we end up spending a lot of our life worrying about things that will never happen and being blasé about things that will.

Fear is the basis of all addictions. It's the force that makes the trap so powerful. Addicts are fooled into believing that they're deriving some form of pleasure or support from the drug. It's ingenious because it works back to front. It's when you're not drinking that you suffer the slightly ill-at-ease, empty, insecure feeling of not being comfortable in your skin. When you drink, you partially relieve that feeling and your brain is fooled into believing that the alcohol is giving you a little boost. In fact, it's alcohol that created the ill-at-ease feeling in the first place. The more you drink, the more it drags you down and the greater you feel the need for what you perceive as your last little crutch.

This is why drinkers can never win while they're in the trap. When you're drinking you wish you didn't have to. It's only when you can't drink that it appears to be so precious. What sort of pleasure is that?

## *ONCE YOU UNDERSTAND THE ALCOHOL TRAP COMPLETELY, YOU WILL HAVE NO MORE NEED OR DESIRE TO DRINK*

## FEAR OF FAILURE

Being addicted to alcohol is like being in a prison. Every aspect of your life is controlled by drinking: your daily routine, your hopes, your view of the world, your suffering. Of course, you're not physically imprisoned. There are no walls or bars. The prison is in your mind. However, as long as you remain a slave to alcohol, you will experience the same psychological symptoms as an inmate locked in a cell.

If you've tried and failed to quit drinking you will know that it leaves you feeling more trapped than you did before you made the attempt. You've seen movies where a prisoner is thrown into a cell and the first thing he does is run to the door and wrench at the handle. This confirms his predicament: He really is locked in.

Trying and failing to quit has the same effect on the addict. It reinforces the belief that you're trapped in a prison from which there is no escape. This can be a crushing experience and many people conclude that the best way to avoid the misery of failure is to avoid trying to escape in the first place. We put off what we regard as the "evil day" because we fear we're going to have to go through some terrible trauma and will probably fail in any case.

Fear keeps us locked in the misery of the addiction and prevents us risking the disappointment of failure. What we don't realize is:

### THE PERSON WHO TUGS AT THE PRISON DOOR AND FINDS IT FIRMLY LOCKED IS SIMPLY USING THE WRONG METHOD OF ESCAPE

The fear of failure is illogical in this case. It's the fear of something that has already happened. You're already a slave. In the case of alcohol addiction, you suffer a compulsion to keep drinking even though it's ruining your life and making you miserable. As long as that continues, you will continue to feel a failure.

When channeled properly, the fear of failure can be a positive force. It's the emotion that focuses the mind of the runner on the starting blocks, the ballerina waiting in the wings, and the student going into an exam. Fear of failure is the little voice in your head that reminds you to prepare thoroughly, to remember everything you've rehearsed and trained for, and leave nothing to chance.

The addict's fear of failure is based on an illusion. In fact, you have nothing to lose by trying, even if you do fail. By not trying, you insure that you remain permanently in the trap. In other words:

### IF YOU SUCCUMB TO THE FEAR OF FAILURE YOU'RE GUARANTEED TO SUFFER THE VERY THING YOU FEAR

But failure isn't the only fear that keeps addicts imprisoned in the trap.

## FEAR OF SUCCESS

It's a sad fact that many long-term prisoners in the penal system reoffend soon after they're released. This depressing tendency occurs not just because they haven't learned the error of their ways, but because in some cases they actually want to go back inside. They yearn for the "security" of the prison. Life on the outside is alien and frightening for them, more frightening than life on the inside. It's unfamiliar and they don't feel equipped to handle it.

The same fear afflicts addicts. They're afraid that they won't be able to enjoy or cope with life without their "crutch," that they'll have to go through some terrible trauma to get free of it and that they'll be condemned to a life of sacrifice and deprivation.

In the case of the person suffering from alcohol addiction, failure means remaining in the old, familiar prison cell; success means coming out into the unknown and that can seem daunting. Like those long-term prisoners, you may be fearful of what life will be like outside and dread the self-discipline, sacrifice, and deprivation that you fear will be waiting for you.

Perhaps you've been tricked into believing that going through life without drinking is boring. Though you're well aware of the misery that your drinking causes, you may now have come to think of it as part of your identity. Perhaps you even regard it with a perverse kind of respect, as if there were some sort of shambolic charisma about it. The Hollywood image of the heavy drinker, the chain-smoker, and the gambler can suggest that it makes us attractive. Heroic characters in books and films are frequently portrayed as having one or more of these characteristics and the implication is that it makes them human, charming, exciting, lovable. To the audience maybe; in real life it makes them miserable and impossible to live with.

## WIN THE TUG-OF-WAR

Cast the illusions aside and be clear in your mind: The panic feeling that makes you afraid even to try to quit drinking is caused by alcohol, not relieved by it. And one of the greatest benefits you'll receive when you quit is never to suffer it again. The tug-of-war of fear is easy to win because one side is made up of illusions. Remove the illusions and, instead of a conflict of will, all your will is going in one direction—away from alcohol.

## TAKE AWAY THE ALCOHOL AND THE FEAR
## GOES TOO

If I could transport you now into your mind and body after you become free with this method, you would think, "Will I really feel this good?"

Fear will have been replaced by elation, despair by optimism, self-doubt by confidence, apathy by dynamism. Your physical health will of course improve radically too. You will enjoy a newfound energy, as well as the ability to truly relax.

Maybe you've tried to stop in the past and gone for weeks, months, even years without drinking, but still found that you missed it. Trust me, this method is different. You will not miss drinking. You're not giving anything up. There is no sacrifice involved. Instead, you're removing something from your life that has made you miserable.

### THERE IS NOTHING TO FEAR

You're trading lack of control over your drinking for total control —no choice for absolute choice.

Part of you feels that alcohol is your friend, your constant companion and support.

Get it clearly into your mind, this is an illusion. Alcohol is your worst enemy and, far from supporting you, it's driving you deeper and deeper into misery. You instinctively know this, so open your mind and follow your instincts.

## REMOVING ALL DOUBTS

Think about all the good things you stand to gain by overcoming your drinking problem. Think of the enormous self-respect you'll have, the time and energy you'll save, not only by taking alcohol out of your life but also by taking out all the covering up, lying to your friends and family, deceiving your workmates, and trying to convince yourself that you're in control.

That little boost you feel every time you succumb to your addiction is a mere hint of how a nondrinker feels all the time, and how you will feel when you're free. Wouldn't you rather feel like that all the time, without any effort or cost, and without the horrible lows that alcohol brings?

If you saw a heroin addict suffering the misery of drug addiction, would you advise them to keep injecting heroin into their veins, rather than try living without that "wonderful high" they experience every time they get a fix? Of course you wouldn't. You would see that the "high" is nothing more than relief from the withdrawal caused by the drug as it leaves the body. It would be obvious to you that the only way to escape the withdrawal permanently would be to stop taking the drug.

Perhaps you don't think you have the same problem as a heroin addict. I can assure you, all addicts are caught in the same trap. See yourself as you would see a heroin addict and give yourself the only logical piece of advice:

### *STOP DRINKING!*

The only reason drinkers fail to see the solution as simple is because they have been brainwashed into the tug-of-war of fear. Once you can see that there is nothing to fear, that you're not giving up anything or depriving yourself in any way, stopping is easy.

So far I have given you three instructions to put you in the right frame of mind so that this book can help you overcome your drinking problem:

1.   Follow all the instructions

2.   Keep an open mind

3.   Begin with a feeling of elation

Drinking does absolutely nothing positive for you whatsoever and the beliefs that have imprisoned you in the alcohol trap are merely illusions. You have everything to gain and nothing to lose by stopping. There is nothing to fear. Life will become infinitely more enjoyable from the moment you become free.

Perhaps you're afraid that the process itself will be painful. You may have struggled to quit before by using willpower and found it a tortuous experience. That's because the willpower method doesn't work. It leaves you feeling deprived and so, as I will explain in the next chapter, you never really get completely free.

It's now time for my fourth instruction:

### NEVER DOUBT YOUR DECISION TO QUIT

I want you to think about everything we've covered so far and be clear that you understand and accept it. If you're struggling with any of the instructions, go back and reread the relevant chapter until it becomes clear. It's essential that you not only follow the instructions but also that you understand them.

Sometimes we meet people who say they understand all the instructions, yet they still retain a desire to drink. They have missed something somewhere along the line and it's essential for them to go back and identify where the problem lies. It's often that they haven't truly opened their mind. If you follow all the instructions, you will no longer feel the desire to drink. Remove the desire and the prison door will spring open.

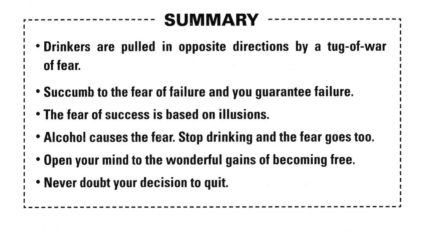

```
┌─────────────────  SUMMARY  ─────────────────┐
│ • Drinkers are pulled in opposite directions by a tug-of-war │
│   of fear.                                                    │
│                                                              │
│ • Succumb to the fear of failure and you guarantee failure.  │
│                                                              │
│ • The fear of success is based on illusions.                │
│                                                              │
│ • Alcohol causes the fear. Stop drinking and the fear goes too. │
│                                                              │
│ • Open your mind to the wonderful gains of becoming free.    │
│                                                              │
│ • Never doubt your decision to quit.                         │
└──────────────────────────────────────────────┘
```

Chapter 9

# WILLPOWER

*If you think you have failed to quit drinking because you lack the willpower, think again.*

If it's easy to quit drinking, why do so many people find it incredibly hard? The reason's simple: They're using the wrong method.

The simplest of tasks becomes difficult if you go about it the wrong way. For example, opening a door. You know how to open a door—you push on the handle and it swings open with the minimum of effort. But have you ever come across a door with no handle and pushed on the wrong side, where the hinges are? You're met with firm resistance. The door might budge a tiny bit, but it won't swing open. It requires a huge amount of effort and determination. Push on the correct side and the door opens without you even having to think about it.

Most drinkers find it difficult to stop because they use the willpower method. It's not their fault. All the received wisdom from governments and health organizations is that you need willpower to quit. Only Easyway takes the opposite view. People who try to quit with the willpower method endure a constant conflict of will, a mental tug-of-war. On one side your rational brain knows you should stop drinking because it's making you ill, affecting your behavior, costing you a fortune, controlling your life, and causing you misery. On the other side your addicted brain makes you panic at the thought of being deprived of your pleasure or support. On the willpower method you focus on all the reasons for stopping and hope you can last long enough without drinking for the desire eventually to go.

The fundamental problem with this is that you still perceive drinking as a pleasure or a support and, therefore, you feel you've made a sacrifice. You force yourself into a self-imposed tantrum, like a child being deprived of its toys. This feeling of deprivation makes you miserable, which in turn makes you want to try to cheer yourself up by doing the one thing you've vowed not to do—have a drink.

You only need willpower to stop if you have a conflict of will. We're going to resolve that conflict by removing one side of the tug-of-war, so that all your will is going against drinking. Using willpower for the rest of your life to try not to drink is unlikely to prove successful and will not make you happy; removing the desire to drink will.

**ALLEN CARR'S EASYWAY REMOVES THE NEED FOR WILLPOWER BY REMOVING THE ILLUSION THAT YOU'RE MAKING A SACRIFICE**

Some people do manage to quit drinking, smoking, gambling, and other addictions through sheer force of will, but they never completely break free of their addiction, as I will explain in a moment. In most cases, the willpower method fails and you end up back in the trap, feeling more helpless and miserable than before.

## *ENCOURAGING SOMEONE TO QUIT THROUGH THE USE OF WILLPOWER IS LIKE TELLING THEM TO OPEN A DOOR BY PUSHING ON THE HINGES*

## HOW WEAK-WILLED ARE YOU?

Just as the willpower method is commonly assumed to be the only way to cure an addiction, those who fail to quit that way and remain in the trap are generally branded as weak-willed. Indeed, they brand themselves as weak-willed. They assume it's they who have failed, not the method.

Perhaps you think that's why you've been unable to quit drinking up until now: because you lack the strength of will. If that's the case, then you haven't yet understood the nature of the trap you're in.

Ask yourself whether you're weak-willed in other ways. Perhaps you're a smoker or you eat too much and you regard these conditions as further evidence of a weak will. There is a connection between all addictions, but the connection is not that they're signs of a lack of willpower. On the contrary, they're more likely evidence of a strong will. What they all share is that they're traps created by misleading information and untruths. And one of the most misleading untruths of all is that quitting requires willpower.

### IN HER OWN WORDS: RACHEL

As the manager of a sports center in the 1980s, I found myself having to fight my corner in a man's world. It could be quite pressurized at times, but I relished the challenge and enjoyed it when I got my way. To be honest, I got my way most of the time. I think some of the men I dealt with were scared of me! But we got on well and often went out drinking together, both for work and socially.

In my late 20s I decided it was time to start a family and the first thing I needed to do was cut down on the drinking. I wanted to be in good health for my baby. I thought it would be easy but as time went by and I couldn't get pregnant I started to console myself with a drink in the evening. Pretty soon that became a drink or two at lunchtime too and before long I was drinking as much as ever.

I went to see the doctor about my inability to get pregnant and she asked me how much I drank. I lied to her, but she was still surprised by my answer and told me I should try to stop. So I did. I tried with all my might, but although I had a very good reason for not drinking,

I just couldn't get the craving for drink out of my mind. I found it really frustrating. I had never had a problem getting my way before and in every other aspect of life, if I turned my mind to something I knew I could achieve it. But when it came to drink, I just seemed to be too weak-willed. I have now quit after going to an Allen Carr's Easyway center and realize that being weak-willed wasn't the problem; it was the belief that I was depriving myself of a genuine pleasure. Because I'm strong-willed, I clung to that belief even more obstinately and forced myself into a corner. The funny thing is that when I quit with Easyway, I didn't need willpower at all and I've never missed alcohol.

It takes a strong-willed person to persist in doing something that goes against all their instincts. You know that drinking is dragging you further and further down, making you increasingly stressed and unhappy, threatening to destroy your relationships, your health, your career, your life, and yet you continue to do it. That is not the behavior of a weak-willed person.

When you organize your life so you can sneak out to buy booze without arousing suspicion; when you get up early in the morning or stay up late at night so you can drink without your family looking over your shoulder; when you borrow money from friends and lie to them about what you need it for; when you sacrifice the pastimes you used to enjoy because your only interest in life is drink… all these actions take a strong will.

If I saw you trying to open a door by pushing on the hinges and I told you you'd find it easier if you pushed on the handle, but you ignored me and insisted on pushing on the hinges, I'd call you willful, not weak-willed.

The ex-con who reoffends soon after being released from prison is not weak-willed; he's showing a strong will to get back inside. It takes real determination to commit a crime.

Think of all the people you know who've had alcohol problems. There are enough high-profile examples to illustrate that problem drinking is not exclusive to the weak-willed. Presidents, captains of industry, movie stars, singers, sports stars, writers... the rehab centers are full of people who have found success and made a name for themselves in such fields. The common ground between them all is that they reached their position through determination and hard work. In other words, they had immense willpower. So why would their willpower fail them in this one area?

I'm sure you too can find evidence that you're strong-willed. How do you react when people tell you that you have to change your ways and sort out your drinking problem? Don't you find you tend to do the opposite? Wouldn't you describe that as willful?

In fact, it tends to be the most strong-willed people who find it hardest to quit by willpower.

Why? Because on the willpower method you force yourself into a self-imposed tantrum like a child being denied its toys. Which child will keep its tantrum going longest and loudest— a weak-willed one or a strong-willed one?

**IN HIS OWN WORDS: JIM**

I quit drinking for nine months once. I threw out every drop of booze in the house and made sure I never walked into a bar. There were times when it took incredible willpower. All the while I clung to the belief that eventually it would get easier.

But after nine months I couldn't stand it any more. That first drink was an enormous relief, but did it make me happy? Not a chance. I cried like a baby. I felt such a failure and I was convinced that I was going to be at the mercy of this addiction for the rest of my life—and that was unlikely to be as long as I'd hoped.

The worst thing was that I felt I'd fallen just short of the line. I honestly thought that I was close to winning the battle, because I had gone so long without a drink. I couldn't understand why I hadn't been able to hold out just that bit longer. But now I understand I was nowhere near the finishing line. The truth is, there was no finishing line. In trying to quit through willpower, I was condemning myself to a lifetime of torture.

When you try to quit by the willpower method, the struggle never ends. As long as you continue to believe that you're giving something up, you will always feel deprived. The stronger your willpower, the longer you will put yourself through the agony. Jim was strong-willed enough to hold out for nine months, but the longer he went on suffering a sense of deprivation, the more powerful his craving for alcohol became.

## CROSSING THE LINE THE EASY WAY

With Easyway, the elation of crossing the finishing line occurs as soon as you remove the fear and illusions and stop drinking. That's when you're free of the addiction that has kept you enslaved. You need to understand that you will NOT get to that line by forcing yourself to suffer.

Suffering does not work. As I explained in Chapter 4, rather than helping you to quit, it actually encourages you to stay hooked because:

1. It reinforces the myth that quitting is hard and, therefore, adds to your fear.

2. It creates a feeling of deprivation, which you will seek to alleviate in your usual way—you will fall back into the trap.

Once you have failed on the willpower method, it's even harder to try again, because, like Jim, you will have reinforced the belief that it's impossible to cure your problem. People who have tried the willpower method and failed will tell you they felt an enormous sense of relief when they gave in and had that first drink. It's important to understand that this relief is nothing more than a temporary end to the self-inflicted pain. They don't think, "Great!

I've fallen back into the alcohol trap." It's not a pleasure. In fact, it's accompanied by feelings of failure and foreboding, guilt, and disappointment.

That first drink after you've tried to quit is not pleasurable at all, despite what others might tell you. They're confusing pleasure with the relief of ending the psychological craving caused by the feeling of deprivation. With Easyway there is no deprivation.

## OTHER QUITTERS

You may know people who are trying to overcome alcoholism or some other addiction by using willpower. You may admire their determination and wish you could do the same. STOP. Remember what I have told you about the willpower method and see things as they really are.

People who try to quit by the willpower method can have a harmful effect on your own desire to quit. They either brag about the sacrifices they're making, or they whine about them. Either way, they reinforce the misconception that quitting involves feeling deprived. It's important that you ignore the advice of anyone who claims to have quit by the willpower method. The beautiful truth is there is no sacrifice.

You're soon to become a happy nondrinker. To do that, you need only to understand that you're not "giving up" anything. You only need willpower if you're caught up in the tug-of-war of fear.

Take away the fear on one side and there is nothing to tug against. It's easy.

Jim was waiting for the moment when the pain ended to

become a happy nondrinker. But there is nothing to wait for. You become a happy nondrinker the moment you unravel all the illusions that have led you into the alcohol trap, free yourself from fear, and stop drinking with a feeling of excitement and elation.

If you've followed me so far and understood that the beliefs that keep you in the alcohol trap are illusions, that you're not required to summon any willpower to stop drinking, and that there is nothing to fear, you should already be feeling excited. You have taken a major step in solving your drink problem.

### *YOU CAN SOON START LIVING YOUR LIFE AGAIN, KNOWING YOU'RE NO LONGER A SLAVE TO ALCOHOL. YOU'LL BE BACK IN CONTROL AND YOU'LL BE FREE*

Isn't that worth celebrating?

There's another obstacle that could be preventing you from feeling this sense of excitement. Not everyone who tries and fails to stop by using the willpower method concludes that they're weak-willed, but rather than confront the true reasons why they remain hooked, they decide it must be down to another aspect of their personality over which they have no control. When all other explanations fail them, there is one theory that conveniently provides all the excuses they need to stay in the trap: the so-called addictive personality.

## SUMMARY

- Quitting is only hard if you use the wrong method.

- Addiction is not a symptom of being weak-willed. In fact, it's often the opposite.

- With the willpower method, you never reach the finishing line.

- People who brag or whine about quitting by willpower still believe they're making a sacrifice.

- With Easyway, you cross the line the moment you reverse the brainwashing and stop drinking.

# THE ADDICTIVE PERSONALITY

*The theory of the addictive personality stems from looking at the situation from the wrong perspective. The character traits shared by addicts are not the cause of their addiction, they're the result.*

People with an alcohol problem tend to feel weak and foolish. In order to combat this feeling, we make up excuses in a vain attempt to explain why we're so helplessly hooked:

"I'm going through a bad time at the moment. I'll stop when things pick up."

"Everyone likes a drink from time to time."

Even when it's pointed out that their problem is an addiction to alcohol, they're ready with the excuse for not quitting:

"I have an addictive personality."

Millions of people throughout the world are suffering from alcohol addiction. When you come out of your cocoon and speak to people about your problems and discover that many of them are experiencing, or have experienced, exactly what you're going through, then you begin to see that the addiction is not a weakness in the individual but a weakness in the society that brainwashes individuals into falling for the trap.

Many addicts believe that there's something in their genetic makeup that makes them more susceptible than most people to becoming hooked, and makes it harder for them to escape. It's a convenient excuse, but all it does is ensure that they remain forever trapped, their suffering increasing, and the misery leading them closer and closer to despair.

Sadly, their misconception is backed up by a number of so-called "experts," who support the theory of the addictive personality. The term is bandied about so often that it's easy to be fooled into believing it's an established condition. It's not. It's a theory, largely based on the incidence of multiple addictions in the same people, e.g. drinkers who are also smokers or gamblers, or heroin addicts who smoke and are heavily in debt.

All these addictions are caused by the same thing, but it's not the personality: It's the misguided belief that the thing you're addicted to gives you a genuine pleasure or support. Remember:

### *THE CRAVING IS NOT RELIEVED BY THE DRUG YOU'RE ADDICTED TO, IT'S CAUSED BY IT*

Remember, the fear of success drives people with a drink problem to seek reasons to avoid even trying to quit. The addictive personality theory gives them the perfect excuse. If you think you have an addictive personality, you will regard quitting as an impossible task. "How can I override my own genetic make-up?" This illusion can also be reinforced by your failed attempts to quit by using willpower.

It's further confirmed by people who have quit by using the willpower method and are feeling deprived because they still believe they're making a sacrifice. After all, if they have abstained for years and are still craving their little crutch, surely there must be some flaw in their genetic makeup that keeps drawing them back?

But there is another explanation, and one that has been proven by Easyway time and time again.

## THE FEAR OF SUCCESS IS BASED ON AN ILLUSION

The illusion is that you're making a genuine sacrifice. In reality, you're not "giving up" anything. People who whine about having quit are constantly tormented because they still believe that they're depriving themselves. Don't be fooled by these illusions. Pleading an addictive personality is just another cop-out. You don't want to stay enslaved by alcohol, with all the fear, misery, and sickness that goes with it; that's why you're reading this book. You have made the decision to escape and you're well on the way to doing just that.

Escape is easy, provided you keep an open mind. If you cling to the excuse that you have an addictive personality, it means that your mind is not open and you risk sentencing yourself to remain enslaved for the rest of your life.

I used to think that my addiction to smoking must be something I'd inherited. I watched my father die of lung cancer and I assumed I would go the same way. To any observer I must have looked like I was happily going to an early grave, puffing on cigarettes all the way. In truth, I was desperate to quit. I was terrified of the threat of lung cancer and a slow, painful death. But I felt stupid and helpless because all my attempts had failed and so putting it down to a flaw in my personality seemed to offer the only rational explanation.

I now know that I was not stupid, that the ingenuity of the trap means that anybody can be conned, and most people are to some extent. But once you understand how addiction works, the illusions disappear, and you realize that you're complete without your little "crutch." With it, you're a slave.

## DEGREES OF ADDICTION

So why do some people fall deeper into the trap than others? Why can one person have the occasional drink, while another ends up reaching for the booze first thing in the morning? Doesn't that suggest that one has an addictive personality and the other doesn't?

It does point to a difference between them, yes, but there are numerous differences between people that can explain why one person's behavior differs from another's in this context, and none of them has anything to do with an addictive personality.

For most people the first experience of drinking is revolting. For some, that's enough to put them off ever drinking again. Others see it as a challenge that must be surmounted if they're to earn respect, and make a point of drinking as much as they can. Others can't afford to drink more than a small amount each week. In addition to that, our behavior is closely linked to the influences we're subjected to as we grow up: different parents, teachers, friends, things we read, watch and listen to, places we go, people we meet, etc.

All these factors will have a bearing on how quickly we descend into the trap. The celebrities that we hear about who seem to fall so rapidly into the trap usually have millions to pour down the drain and the time and opportunity to do so.

## AN AFFINITY BETWEEN WEAKNESSES

You will no doubt have noticed how you and other problem drinkers seem to be a different breed from everyone else. You appear to share similar character traits: an unstable temperament, which swings between exuberance and irritability, a tendency towards excess, a high susceptibility to stress, evasiveness, anxiety, and insecurity.

The temptation is to believe that these character traits are evidence of the addictive personality that led to you having a drink problem. The reality is that they're the result of drinking.

The reason addicts feel more comfortable in the company of similar addicts is not because they're more interesting or fun; on the contrary, the attraction lies in the very fact that they won't challenge you or make you think twice about your addiction, because they're in the same boat. All addicts know that they're doing something stupid and self-destructive. If they're surrounded by other people doing the same thing, they don't feel quite so foolish.

The good news is that, once you're free from the addiction, you also get free from the harmful effects it has on your character.

### THE EVIDENCE OF HISTORY

If there were a gene that predisposed people to become addicts, you would expect the percentage of addicts in the world to have remained fairly constant throughout history. Yet this is not the case. Take smoking: In the 1940s more than 80 percent of the U.K. adult male population was hooked on nicotine; today it's fewer than 25 percent. A similar trend is evident throughout most of Western Europe and North America. So are we to conclude that the proportion of people with addictive personalities has fallen by a whopping 55 percent in just over half a century?

At the same time, the number of smokers in Asia has soared. What complex genetic anomaly is this that rises and falls so rapidly, and even appears to transfer itself wholesale from one continent to another?

## EFFECT NOT CAUSE

It's essential that you understand that you didn't become addicted to alcohol because you have an addictive personality. If you think you have an addictive personality, it's simply because you got addicted to alcohol.

This is the trick that addiction plays on you. It makes you feel that you're dependent on your addiction and that there's some weakness in your character or genetic makeup. It distorts your perceptions and thereby maintains its grip on you.

The addictive personality theory encourages the belief that escape is out of your hands and that you're condemned to a life of slavery and misery.

Remember, you didn't feel the need or desire to drink until you started. It was drinking that created the addiction, not the other way around.

This slavery will soon be behind you. Once you can strip away the illusions and see the situation in its true light, you'll wonder how you were ever conned into seeing it differently. Like millions of people around the world, you have been the victim of an ingenious trap. Recognize the trap for what it is, dismiss the idea of a flaw in your personality, and you will be ready to walk free.

### BINGE MISERY

Have you ever opened a box of chocolates with the intention of only eating one, and found yourself ten minutes later having devoured the lot? Why do we do it? There is no pleasure in it. Logic would suggest that if one chocolate tastes divine, a whole box should be an earthshattering experience, but the reality is nothing like that, is it? Physically you feel bloated and sick, while emotionally you feel disgusted with yourself and horribly out of control.

Drinkers can get into a similar frenzy. Remember David's story on page 15? He would drink endlessly for days, until all the drink had run out. When he came around and saw what he had done, he felt disgusted with himself.

Just as you don't savor each chocolate, you don't stop to savor each drink. In fact there's nothing to savor. One drink leads to the next, and the next, and the next, and the further you go without achieving fulfillment, the more frenzied and ridiculous the drinking becomes. Like a dog chasing its tail, you go faster and faster chasing something you can never attain.

This is typical of addictive behavior. People often claim that they drink to be sociable, yet they often binge on their own, where nobody can see what they themselves regard as shameful.

The Big Monster tells you that alcohol is the only thing that can fill the void—but it's alcohol that creates the void. You experience a triple low: a physical low caused by a combination of withdrawal and the damage alcohol does to your body, a psychological craving and the sheer misery of being an addict.

This triple low becomes your new idea of normal.

The Little Monster itself is easy to deal with. The edgy feeling caused by alcohol withdrawal involves no pain and, provided you follow the instructions I will give you later, it's no problem when you stop. The real trouble with the Little Monster in the body is that it triggers the Big Monster in the mind and the mental craving of "I want a drink."

If you then can't have a drink, you feel uptight, frustrated, and deprived. It's like having an itch that you're not allowed to scratch. If you have something else occupying your mind, you may not even be aware of it, so the physical aggravation is hardly perceptible. But once you become aware of it and want to scratch it but can't, the mental torture can become unbearable as you're not allowed to do the one thing that you know will give you relief. However, in the case of alcohol, it's the alcohol that's causing the itch. The beauty of Easyway is that it removes the Big Monster in the mind, so that you don't feel frustrated or deprived when you quit. Killing off the Little Monster in the body then becomes easy.

## FIX FIXATION

It's revealing that addicts use the word "fix." A fix is a solution to a problem; you fix something that is broken. When something breaks and you fix it, it's never quite as good as it was originally. A fix is not an improvement. It's not a pleasure or reward. It's nothing more than relief, like taking off tight shoes.

## ACCEPTANCE

All problem drinkers want to quit. At the same time they're afraid to "give up" their little pleasure or support. This conflict leaves them feeling helpless and stupid. They don't understand why they can't just take control of the situation and sort themselves out.

As a result, they tend to bury their head in the sand and pretend that they don't have a problem. They lie to themselves about the state they're in and pretend that they're in control. The beautiful truth is that all drinkers can take control any time they want to.

All they have to do is stop drinking. It's as easy as that, provided they understand the trap they're in and follow the right method to escape.

You have already taken a big step. You have overcome denial and accepted that you have a drink problem. That's why you're reading this book. That is another big step. You have taken action to do something about the problem. Now all you have to do is kill the Big Monster. Once the Big Monster is dead, you will find it easy to cut off the supply to the Little Monster and it will die very quickly.

You kill the Big Monster by removing the illusions that create the desire to drink. Think about how those illusions were created and who by.

The parents, friends, and other role models who all brainwashed you into believing that drinking is a pleasure and a support were all brainwashed themselves.

I have explained how alcohol gives no genuine pleasure or support; it merely creates the illusion. Your belief in pleasure is what put you in the trap. Now that you understand the nature of the trap, you can see that there is no genuine pleasure. You understand that alcohol does not fill the void; it creates it.

## YOU HAVE ALREADY BEGUN TO KILL THE BIG MONSTER

Congratulations! You have come a long way toward curing your drink problem and it's essential that you're not diverted from your path. There are several things that could hinder your escape. Perhaps there is a part of you that still believes you get some pleasure or support from drinking. Perhaps you're afraid that life without alcohol will leave you feeling deprived in some way. There are many influences out there that can mislead you with false ideas like these, and some of them are well-meaning. Please take note of my next instruction:

## IGNORE ALL ADVICE AND INFLUENCES THAT CONFLICT WITH EASYWAY

The truth is you're not "giving up" anything. Instead, you're freeing yourself from a trap that has been causing you misery and threatening your wellbeing and everything you value. It's time to rejoice. The Big Monster is dying and soon you will be ready to kill the Little Monster too.

## SUMMARY

• The addictive personality is a myth that gives the addict an excuse to avoid even trying to escape.

• The personality traits shared by addicts are caused by their addiction; they're not the cause.

• Be aware of the two monsters: the Little Monster that cries out for alcohol and the Big Monster that interprets its cries as "I want a drink."

Chapter 11

# NORMAL DRINKERS

## IN THIS CHAPTER
*• THE BENEFITS OF ALCOHOL  • CUTTING DOWN*
*• DIFFERENT STAGES OF THE SAME DISEASE*
*• THE JOYS OF "NORMAL" DRINKING*

*Do you want to quit completely or merely cut down on the amount you drink?*

We have established that problem drinking has nothing to do with an addictive personality or a lack of willpower but is caused by illusions that trap us in a prison of fear. You may be wondering, then, why you can't keep your drinking to a controlled level, like all those happy "normal" drinkers.

All drinkers believe they get some pleasure or support from drinking. That means 90 percent of the adult population believe that alcohol benefits them in some way.

A common conversation we have with people who come to us with a drink problem goes like this:

They begin by asking, "Do you ever want a drink?"

"Never."

"Do you think you could have an occasional drink and not get hooked again?"

"What would be the point, since I have no desire to drink alcohol?"

"Could you teach me to have an occasional drink without getting hooked again?"

"I'm teaching you how to remove the desire to consume alcohol at all. Why would you want to have an occasional drink? Would you want to take an occasional dose of arsenic?"

"Why on Earth would I want to do that?"

"Exactly."

At this point a look of realization usually comes over them. They've begun the conversation with the suggestion that alcohol provides some benefit. I've ended it by highlighting that alcohol is neither a pleasure nor a support; it's an addictive poison, pure and simple. When the client accepts this, the fear they have about never drinking again—the fear of success—disappears.

This is a wonderful feeling, a revelation, like the sun appearing from behind a cloud. Or when you see the hidden message in an illusion, like the STOP diagram. Just by seeing the facts in a new light, you go from fear to joy in an instant.

FEAR: I WILL NEVER BE ABLE TO DRINK AGAIN.

JOY: I NEVER HAVE TO DRINK AGAIN.

I've talked a lot about the disadvantages of alcohol. For the sake of balance, it's only fair that I tell you what its advantages are. There are three things:

- An anesthetic
- A detergent and antiseptic
- A fuel

Similar to meths, in fact. Would you drink meths and believe it was doing you good? Now remind yourself of what you know about alcohol:

- A powerful poison—half a pint drunk neat will kill you
- A highly addictive drug
- A drain on your finances—an average drinker spends more than $75,000
- It impedes judgment and concentration
- It weakens your immune system
- It destroys your nervous system
- It causes stress
- It tastes foul

Alcohol is also a diuretic. Diuretics make you thirsty. That's why after a binge you wake at 3 a.m. with a mouth like a dry riverbed, and one thing on your mind: water! If alcohol quenched thirst the last thing you would need, after all that liquid, is even more. The fact that some people can drink 16 pints of beer proves alcohol creates thirst: you couldn't drink 16 pints of water if you tried!

Like all addictive drugs, alcohol creates withdrawal and then—as you develop tolerance—ceases fully to relieve it. So you want more. On top of that there's the fact that it creates thirst while seeming to quench it. The water content slakes your thirst immediately. So your brain is fooled into believing alcohol quenches thirst. But once the alcohol content is absorbed, it makes you thirstier, so that's another reason you soon want more and with each subsequent drink you just get thirstier and thirstier.

Now, why would you feel miserable about never drinking alcohol again? It does absolutely nothing for you but damages you in all these ways. Wouldn't it be wonderful never to have to drink again?

So why do we envy those "normal" drinkers who haven't had their life ruined by alcohol? Well, for that very reason alone, you might say. But then why not envy a nondrinker? They haven't had their life ruined by alcohol either. If you think it's better to be a "normal" drinker than a nondrinker, that's because you still believe there is some benefit to drinking.

You also believe that the "normal" drinker is in control. That's the difference between them and you: While drinking controls you, they seem to be able to decide when they drink and how much, without any trouble at all. But is that really the case? Remember, all drinkers try very hard to give the impression that they're in control.

The fly on the upper slope of the pitcher plant thinks it's in control. It knows it can fly away at any moment. But it doesn't. It continues to drink, sliding further and further into the plant, until it's too late and the fly is doomed. Anyone observing this will know that the fly is doomed the moment it lands on the lip of the plant. The same inevitable process follows time after time. The fly is never in control. It's controlled by the pitcher plant from the moment it picks up the scent of the nectar.

A similar scenario is acted out in the Hitchcock movie *Notorious*. The heroine is ill and is being nursed by her husband.

Then she discovers that she's not really ill, he's poisoning her. She tries to escape, but the drug is having a debilitating effect on her legs and leaving her mind addled. Ring any bells?

Alcohol isn't the drug being used in the movie, but the comparison is frighteningly apt. While she thinks she's being nursed by her husband, she has no fear of the food he's giving her. She thinks it's doing her good. "Normal" drinkers have no fear of alcohol for the same reason. Like the heroine, and like the fly on the upper slope of the pitcher plant, they're oblivious to the danger they're in. By the time the true situation is revealed and fear kicks in, they're way beyond the point where they lost control.

The crucial difference is that the person administering the poison is you. Unlike the fly or the heroine in the movie, you have the power to stop.

Let's look at another scenario. Imagine you have a spot on your face. Someone gives you an ointment that they say will clear it up, so you rub it on and sure enough the spot disappears. A week later the spot's back, only bigger and redder this time. You apply more ointment and it disappears again. Five days later, it's back, but now it's more than just a spot, it's a rash. As you go on, the duration between the rash breaking out becomes shorter and shorter and it becomes bigger and itchier each time. Imagine the horror you'd feel, knowing that it's going to get worse and worse until you can find a cure. You're also so reliant on that bottle of ointment that you're prepared to pay a fortune for it and you're afraid to go anywhere without it.

Then you discover that you're not the only one suffering this problem. Millions of other people are in exactly the same boat, all handing over a fortune to the ointment industry. And so your nightmare continues, until one day you meet a man who says he used to suffer from the same problem but solved it. You ask him his secret and he says, "Oh, I realized the ointment was causing the rash so I stopped using it." He advises you to do the same— the rash will clear up in a few days and you'll never suffer it again.

What would you do? Would you feel miserable that you could never use the ointment again, or would you be elated that you never had to? Now apply this logic to alcohol. You have the power to free yourself. Isn't that a wonderful feeling?

To the problem drinker, all "normal" drinkers appear to be in control. But would you say a pilot was in control if he was flying through a mountain range with inaccurate charts and his instruments had been tampered with?

He might have his hand on the joystick, but each decision he made would be based on false information. He would be unaware of the danger and so would have no fear, but that doesn't mean the danger isn't there.

## CUTTING DOWN MAKES YOU EVEN MORE MISERABLE

We continue to drink because we're addicted to a drug that controls us. We drink purely and simply to get the alcohol.

When you cut down, you resist the craving for alcohol

between drinks. What effect do you think that has on your desire for alcohol? Imagine I forced you to go without food for a day, how would that affect your desire to eat? Say I starved you for two days, three days, or more—the longer you went without food, the greater your desire for food would become, to the point where you would relish anything I put in front of you.

Hunger is a natural instinct designed for our survival, whereas the Little Monster is a parasite that causes our destruction, but in some ways they are very similar. The longer we go without relieving them, the greater our desire to do so. We all know the meaning of forbidden fruit. The more you cut down on alcohol, the more precious the next drink seems to you. And the more you deny yourself a drink, the more miserable you become.

You try not to give in to the cravings because another part of your brain is feeling rather pleased with itself for apparently taking control of the situation. This creates a schizophrenic dialogue in your mind, rather like Gollum in *The Hobbit*. One part of your brain is whining about not being able to drink, another is maintaining a haughty superiority as it controls the rations. The result is a constant gabble, dominating your mind with thoughts of your next drink.

## BEING DOMINATED BY ALCOHOL AND BEING IN CONTROL OF IT ARE DIRECT OPPOSITES

At the same time as your desire for alcohol is increasing, something else is taking place. Because you're reducing the dose of poison and the money you spend on booze, the ill effects are waning. But it's these ill effects that made you want to cut down in the first place. Therefore, as your desire increases, you start to forget your reasons for cutting down. Small wonder that most attempts to cut down end up with drinkers eventually returning to their previous intake and more often than not surpassing it.

## CUTTING DOWN REINFORCES THE BELIEF THAT WE CANNOT ENJOY LIFE WITHOUT ALCOHOL

Drinkers who try to cut down are creating a number of serious problems for themselves:

1. They keep themselves addicted to alcohol.

2. They wish their lives away waiting for the next drink.

3. Instead of relieving the craving, whenever they feel like it they force themselves to fight it and so are permanently restless and uptight.

4. They reinforce the illusion that drinking is enjoyable.

When you drink heavily, you lose the illusion of pleasure. Each drink becomes automatic and subconscious. You will find that the occasions when you relish drinking most occur after a period of abstinence. This is because there is no genuine pleasure whatsoever in drinking. All that drinkers enjoy is the ending of the aggravation caused by the craving for alcohol, which nondrinkers do not suffer from in any case.

Cutting down increases the illusion of pleasure because the longer you endure the craving, the greater the sense of pleasure when you relieve it.

If you think increasing the illusion of pleasure sounds like a good thing, think again. The only way to increase the illusion of pleasure is to increase the aggravation. It's like wearing tighter and tighter shoes in order to get increasing relief from taking them off. No drinker, including "normal" drinkers, enjoys the aggravation caused by alcohol. There is a constant impulse to scratch the itch, and the more you scratch it, the worse it gets.

That's why cutting down is unsustainable and usually results in drinking more than before.

## A LIFELONG STRUGGLE

Perhaps you believe there is an idyllic alternative to being either a nondrinker or a problem drinker—a third way: the happy casual drinker. In that case, let me ask you a question: Why are you not one already? And if you claim to be one, why are you reading this book? Let's establish whether you really want to be a casual drinker.

If I said I could fix it so that you could drink just once a week for the rest of your life, would you accept it? Better still, suppose I told you you could control your drinking so that you did it only when you really wanted to? That's a pretty exciting offer, isn't it?

But that's what you already do!

Has anyone ever forced you to drink? Every time you've had a drink you've done so because you wanted to, even though part of your brain wished you didn't.

So I take it that you'll settle for just the one drink a week. Well, if that's what you want, you can do just that. Who's to stop you? In fact, why haven't you just had one drink a week for the whole of your drinking life? Could it be that you wouldn't have been happy drinking just once a week?

Of course you wouldn't. Nor is any other drinker. Agreed, there are drinkers who can discipline themselves to just once a week, but can you really believe that any of them are happy restricting themselves almost every day, for the whole of their lives?

## THE TENDENCY IS TO DRINK MORE, NOT LESS

If you like something and you think it gives you support, why restrict the amount you do it? OK, money plays a part and there'll be times when you're in a place where drinking is forbidden. Then there's the effect you know it will have on those around you; it doesn't look good being drunk at work, or drinking as you walk around shopping.

There are many external forces that restrict the amount you can drink, but if all the restrictions were removed, most drinkers would become heavy drinkers.

My question to the casual drinker is this: "What's the point in drinking at all? Do you think you're getting some genuine pleasure or support from those occasions when you drink?

"If so, why wait so long in between?"

The truth is that most casual drinkers are usually suppressing the urge to drink more. They're still laboring under the illusion that drinking is an escape and a relief. All it takes is a crisis for them to increase their drinking in the belief that it will provide some comfort.

At our centers, we meet people who have become alcoholics in their 30s or 40s or even later, and it doesn't take long to establish that they have spent their entire lives believing that drinking could give them some pleasure or support. The only reason they didn't get hooked sooner was because their desire had never been enough to outweigh their knowledge of the dangers. One trauma was enough to tip the balance.

## DIFFERENT STAGES OF THE SAME DISEASE

It's illogical to believe that there is a fundamental difference between one kind of drinker and another, between "normal" drinkers and problem drinkers. We've established that the problem is not with the alcoholic but with the alcohol. How can the same drug be beneficial for one group of people and devastating for another?

The obvious answer is that alcohol is not beneficial for anybody, and once you strip away the veneer of happiness and control from "normal" drinkers, this becomes abundantly clear. There is no demarcation line between "normal" drinking and problem drinking; it's all part of the same disease. The problem drinker is just at a more advanced stage.

Say you have a tile missing from your roof and rain is dripping in. All you have to do is replace the tile and the problem is solved, immediately and permanently. It will take a little time to clear up the mess, but you will find this clear-up process much easier now that the leak has been repaired.

You can cure a drink problem just as easily by stopping the flow of alcohol. As soon as you do, you know your problem is solved and you can enjoy the process of repairing the damage.

But say you don't replace the roof tile and choose instead just to put buckets under the drip. You might be preventing damage to the interior of your house, but yout have the constant headache of having to empty buckets and replace them. How long are you prepared to do this for?

Do you expect the hole in the roof to just heal over one day? Of course it won't. In fact, sooner or later another tile is blown away and the hole doubles in size. Now you're struggling to catch all the drips and your buckets are overflowing before you can empty them. As time goes on the flow of water gets heavier and heavier and the damage to your house is becoming disastrous. But you can make it stop any time you want, simply by fixing the roof.

Now, would it be logical for a person with two tiles missing to think, "I wish I had one tile missing." Wouldn't they be better off fixing the roof completely? The person with one tile missing is suffering with the same problem as the person with two; it just hasn't reached the disaster stage. But it's only a matter of time.

## THE JOYS OF "NORMAL" DRINKING

"Normal" drinkers like to make out that they're in complete control of their alcohol intake.

"I can take it or leave it."

Why not leave it then? Because they believe that it gives them some pleasure or support and that life would not be as enjoyable without it. Present them with the prospect of life without alcohol and see the panic set in.

I used to go on vacation with a friend and we would always celebrate our arrival with a bottle of champagne on the terrace overlooking the sea. When I told him I had stopped drinking, his first reaction was disappointment. "We'll never be able to enjoy that ritual again," he moped.

He was wrong. The next time we went on vacation we sat out on our first night and shared a drink just as before and I enjoyed it as much as ever. Of course I did: The weather was superb, the view was spectacular, I was with one of my closest friends, and it was the first day of the vacation. It made no difference that I was drinking fruit juice without any poison in it.

But his enjoyment was diminished. He wasn't sure whether I'd mind him drinking alcohol in front of me and he seemed uncomfortable every time I topped up his glass. He clearly regarded my situation as something to be treated delicately, as if I had some sort of terrible disease. The irony is I'd gotten rid of one!

This goes back to the illusion that alcohol is essential for happy occasions. I can think of numerous social occasions that have been ruined by booze, through fights, accidents, people saying and doing stupid things, people getting sick. I can also think of many happy occasions where the company, the setting, the weather, or the food all contributed, but I can't think of a single one when everyone came away raving about the quality of the alcohol.

My friend eventually relaxed and enjoyed our vacation ritual, but I wonder if he would have if I had insisted he didn't drink. Given his attitude to my not drinking, I very much doubt that he could "take it or leave it" on that occasion.

Observe the "normal" drinker when the question of who's going to drive arises. I've witnessed so many discussions between partners who regard themselves as "normal" drinkers.

"Am I driving tonight, darling?"

"I will if you want. I don't mind."

"Really? Are you sure it's not my turn?"

"I can't remember. I don't mind, honestly. I'll drive, you enjoy yourself."

"Well, if you insist. I think I will."

I find these conversations fascinating for several reasons. First, the opening question, "Am I driving tonight, darling?" is cleverly designed to receive the answer "no." But the partner doesn't come back with a straightforward "no," he throws the responsibility back on her: "I will if you want." Then he adds, "I don't mind," meaning, "I'd rather not, but I'll stomach it."

She then expresses her relief by faking surprise at his gallantry. "Really?" Then offers him the chance to change his mind: "Are you sure it's not my turn?" Of course, for him to say, "Yes, it's your turn," would be extremely ungallant, so he feigns ignorance:

"I can't remember." Then he repeats the plaintive "I don't mind", hoping she'll take pity on him and feel guilty, and rubs it in with "you enjoy yourself," implying that there's no chance of enjoying oneself without drinking. She reaffirms this with, "I think I will," and the first thing she does is top up her glass. She can't wait to relieve her craving.

Throughout the conversation, both partners are like prisoners drawing lots for the gallows. Neither wants to come across as so desperate to drink that they'll say, "You drive, I really have to drink tonight," yet the relief of the one and the despondency of the other when it's all resolved is plain to see.

## EXCUSES NOT REASONS

"Normal" drinkers harbor the illusion of pleasure more than problem drinkers. But ask them to define the pleasure and they can't. Instead, they offer defensive excuses:

"I can take it or leave it."

"I don't drink that much."

"It's not doing me any harm."

If they genuinely enjoy a drink, why would they choose to leave it? The only possible reason is that it's causing them a problem. It's common practice to abstain from drinking throughout January, ostensibly to "detox" after the heavy drinking of Christmas.

What are these abstainers trying to prove?

That drink isn't a problem for them.

What are they actually proving?

That it is.

If they didn't think their drinking was a problem and they genuinely enjoyed it, why go without for a whole month? Imagine if a friend told you they were giving up bananas for January. Would you think, "There's someone who's in control of their bananas?" Or would you think, "Golly! I didn't know he had a banana problem!"

As for the excuse, "It's not doing me any harm," even if that were true, is it any reason for doing something? Wearing a top hat and singing "Waltzing Matilda" doesn't do any harm, but I wouldn't choose to do it for that reason. If I did, you'd think I was crazy. But it's not half as crazy as giving the excuse that you drink because it doesn't do you any harm, when everybody knows it does!

I began this chapter with a question: Cut down or quit completely? I hope you can now see that cutting down is not an option. The only way to stop the rain coming in is to repair the hole in the roof. Quitting completely is the only way to free yourself from the alcohol trap.

## SUMMARY

- Alcohol can be used as an antiseptic, a detergent, an anesthetic and a fuel. It has no other benefits at all.
- Cutting down increases the craving.
- Casual drinkers are constantly restricting themselves.
- "Normal" drinking and problem drinking are just different stages of the same disease.

# CHAPTER 12

# CONSUMING QUESTIONS

## IN THIS CHAPTER

• *WHEN DO I BECOME A NONDRINKER?*

• *HOW WILL I KNOW WHEN I'VE HAD MY LAST DRINK?*

• *WILL I EVER BE COMPLETELY FREE?* • *CAN I ENJOY LIFE WITHOUT DRINKING?* • *HOW WILL I COPE IN A CRISIS?*

*As you enter the final stages before becoming a nondrinker, you may still have some lingering concerns. It's time to remove any traces of uncertainty.*

If I took you up in an airplane and told you I wanted you to parachute out, you'd feel a lot better about it if you'd been through a proper course of instruction and you knew and understood everything you had to do. If you've followed everything in this book so far, that's how you should feel now about stopping drinking.

You're about to experience an exhilarating sense of freedom. That's what you were hoping for when you boarded the plane and that's what I've prepared you for. You should feel confident about your every move. But it's completely understandable that, as you stand by the door of the plane, looking out at this wonderful new experience that awaits you, you feel the butterflies in your stomach and a little knot of apprehension.

For the parachutist, these fears are irrational. Millions of people have done it before, the whole process has been tested, you've been given all the instruction you need, and you know it works. All you have to do is jump. Yet the butterflies are completely natural.

The same is true of any lingering concerns you might have about becoming a nondrinker. Even though there is no foundation for these concerns, it would be foolish to suggest they don't exist. It's human nature to feel apprehensive about experiencing something new, even when that experience could be the best thing that's ever happened to you.

## WHEN WILL I KNOW I'VE KICKED IT?

Problem drinkers wish they didn't drink but are also afraid that they will have to go through some terrible ordeal in order to quit, or that life will never be enjoyable again without alcohol. Even though they know that drinking is making them miserable, these fears cause them to put off what they see as the evil day. "I will stop, just not right now."

It's no surprise that we have these fears. All our lives we're led to believe that drinking is a pleasure and a support and that addictions like alcoholism are incurable. These myths are ingrained among our beliefs before we even start to drink. No wonder we find it difficult to believe that stopping can be easy.

Having reached this far in the book, you deserve a pat on the back for following the instructions and making a positive move to end your drinking problem. You'll be eager to get to the end and experience this exhilarating sense of freedom that I keep promising, but how will you know when you've achieved your goal? When will you be able to tell that you've definitely become a nondrinker?

- When you can go a whole day without drinking?
- When you can go a week?
- When you can enjoy social events without alcohol?

All these suggestions assume that you will start off with a feeling of sacrifice or deprivation. If you do, there's no telling how long that feeling will last. The truth is much more straightforward:

## YOU BECOME A NONDRINKER AS SOON AS YOU FINISH YOUR FINAL DRINK

It's not the one you think will be your last, or the one you hope will be your last; when you quit with Easyway there is no doubt and there is no need to wait.

The only way you might regard your final drink with uncertainty is if you fail to follow all the instructions, or you use the willpower method.

## BELIEVING IS SUCCEEDING

Get it clearly into your mind: You won't miss drinking and you will enjoy life more and be better equipped to cope with stress when you're free.

**WHERE THERE'S A WILL, THERE'S A WAIT**

People who quit with the willpower method are always waiting for some sign of confirmation that they're free. They also spend their time suspecting that there could be bad news lurking just around the corner. It's like a dark shadow stalking their every move.

Imagine going for medical tests because you suspect you might have a terminal disease, and being told that you will have to wait months or years for the result. It would be torture—hoping for good news, fearing bad news, and spending every day worrying because you simply don't know for certain which it will be. Now imagine you had to wait the rest of your life for those results. That's what it's like for people who are not certain they've kicked drinking completely. They are waiting for something that they hope will never happen.

This is why the willpower method makes people so miserable. They have to endure the rest of their lives waiting for nothing to happen. It's hardly surprising the vast majority fail.

## IS IT POSSIBLE TO BE CURED COMPLETELY?

Different people reach this stage of the book in different frames of mind. Some think they understand everything and feel certain they're ready to quit.

If that's you, I'm delighted, but let's not jump the gun.

If you're still uncertain, don't worry, all will become clear. Whatever your current frame of mind, take the time and care to read right to the end of the book.

It's perfectly understandable that so many drinkers believe that stopping drinking will be incredibly hard. There is nothing stupid or unusual in that belief. We're subjected to this brainwashing all our lives and then we reinforce it by trying to quit by using the willpower method. All your failed attempts to quit or cut down simply serve to reinforce the belief that stopping requires a superhuman effort.

That desperate craving you get when you're fighting the desire to drink may conflict with everything you know about the evils of alcohol, but the craving is still very real and so is the irritability and misery you feel when you use willpower to try to stop.

As addicts, we find ourselves in a state of confusion. When we're forced to consider drinking logically, we can easily see that it's a fool's game, yet we still feel a desire to do it and this creates an inner tension.

The fact that we can't put our finger on what precise pleasure alcohol gives us only serves to increase the confusion.

The truth is very simple:
- The desire to drink comes from the Big Monster—the illusion that drinking gives us pleasure or support.
- The edgy feeling we get when we're without a drink is merely the Little Monster wanting to be fed.
- The Little Monster was created by drinking in the first place.
- Therefore drinking does not relieve the anxiety, it causes it.

Once you have this clearly in your mind, it's easy to see that if you remove the cause of the anxiety you will immediately start to enjoy life free from drinking.

The willpower method is all about fighting through the anxiety, not removing it. In the first few days after quitting, when your willpower is at its strongest, you may have the upper hand in the battle. But over time your resolve is likely to weaken, the uncertainty sets in and the craving increases.

Now your mind is torn in two, one half determined to be a nondrinker, the other urging you to drink. Is it surprising that we get so confused, irritable, and miserable on the willpower method? It would be a miracle if we didn't!

Even if you starve the Little Monster to death, without destroying the Big Monster you will remain forever vulnerable to the temptation to drink.

With Easyway, you kill the Big Monster first. You unravel the brainwashing and see alcohol for what it really is: an addictive poison that controls and debilitates those who take it. Then the Little Monster is easy to deal with. In fact, you can enjoy the process, confident in the knowledge that you're destroying a mortal enemy.

> **JUST THE ONE**
> Unless you destroy the Big Monster—the desire to drink – you remain forever vulnerable to temptation. That's why AA is right when it tells its clients they're never

cured from alcoholism. With AA's method it's true. As long as the temptation remains, there will always be the danger of slipping back into the trap.

A question we're often asked is, "Once I'm cured, will I be able to have the odd glass?" The answer is simple: "Why would you want to?" If you approach your final drink still thinking that you'd like to have the odd drink now and again, you haven't followed all the instructions and the Big Monster still lurks in your mind.

There will be times when you're tested. Other drinkers who don't understand the alcohol trap will see how confident and in control you are as a nondrinker and will assume the odd one won't set you back. What these drinkers don't understand is that you have absolutely no desire to have just the one. But you understand it.

With AA or the willpower method, you're told that one drink is all it will take to trip you up and throw you back into the pit. AA is correct. The point is with Easyway, you have no more desire to have one drink than you do to take arsenic.

## CAN I ENJOY LIFE WITHOUT DRINKING?

All drinkers fear that if they take drinking out of their life they will take out the enjoyment too. It's easy to see why such a belief would stop anyone from trying to quit. Nobody wants to lead a life of sackcloth and ashes, devoid of pleasure or excitement.

The truth is, drinking actually reduces your ability to derive enjoyment or excitement from anything. It debilitates your senses, plays havoc with your judgment, makes you crushingly dull, vulnerable and insecure, and often results in you being sick.

## IF YOU WANT TO ENJOY LIFE TO THE FULL, SURELY IT'S BETTER TO REMAIN LUCID AND ALERT AND HAVE YOUR BODY FUNCTIONING AT FULL CAPACITY

The brainwashing causes drinkers to have a romanticized image of drinking. Where there have been enjoyable situations involving alcohol, a quick analysis of all the details of that situation will reveal there were other aspects that made it enjoyable: good company, good food, an attractive setting, entertainment, a happy occasion.

If you can think of occasions like this that you consider to have been enjoyable because you were drinking, consider them carefully and try to understand why the drinking appeared to enhance the situation. It doesn't take much to see that in reality it does the opposite. Instead of perpetuating the illusion that such occasions won't be enjoyable again without drinking, remind yourself that you will now be able to enjoy those situations more because you'll be free from three tyrants: the debilitating effects of alcohol, the restlessness of always craving a drink, and the misery of knowing you're an addict.

Most of the time we're not even aware of how alcohol makes us feel. The only time we're really aware of it is when we want to drink but can't, or we're drinking but wishing we didn't have to. In both cases it makes us miserable.

## HOW WILL I COPE IN A CRISIS?

Just as drinkers believe they get pleasure from alcohol, they also believe it provides some sort of support. This is because they tend to turn to drink in times of stress and regard it as a relief.

There are many stressful situations from which you might see drinking as an escape: a family row, pressure at work, even financial problems. You can take yourself away, gaze into the bottom of a glass, and put your problems out of your mind.

But sooner or later you have to return to the real world and, surprise, surprise, the problems are still there. In fact, they've usually gotten worse.

If you believe that alcohol provides a support in these situations, what happens the next time such a situation arises after you've quit? Your brain will tell you, "At times like this I would have had a drink." And you will feel deprived that you can no longer do so.

Think about it: Have you ever found yourself in the midst of a domestic row and thought, "It doesn't matter that we're shouting horrible things at one another and it's really painful because I can just go and have a drink and it will be all right?"

Or did the fact that you drink make the row worse?

Nondrinkers also have to deal with stress, but they're not left moping because they can't drink. All you have to do is accept that, like all nondrinkers, you will have ups and downs in your life after you've quit, and understand that if you start wishing you could drink in such situations, you will be moping for an illusion and creating a void.

## *ALCOHOL REDUCES YOUR ABILITY TO COPE WITH STRESSFUL SITUATIONS AND ADDS TO THE STRESS*

Anticipate the difficult times in life after you've quit and prepare yourself mentally so that you don't get caught out. Remind yourself that any stress you feel is not because you can't drink. Tell yourself, "OK, today is not so great, but at least I haven't got the added problem of being a slave to booze. I'm stronger now." You will find that the stressful situations in your life will actually feel less severe once you're free.

## *BEING FREE ENHANCES ALL SITUATIONS IN LIFE— GOOD AND BAD*

## SUMMARY

- **You become a nondrinker the moment you finish your final drink.**
- **Remove the illusions, kill the Big Monster, win the tug-of-war.**
- **Drinking reduces your ability to make the most of enjoyable occasions.**
- **Drinking doesn't relieve stress; it causes it.**
- **Being free enhances both the ups and the downs.**

# Chapter 13

# NOTHING TO FEAR

## IN THIS CHAPTER
•*RECOGNIZING GENUINE PLEASURES*
•*WHAT YOU'VE ACHIEVED SO FAR* •*TIME TO MAKE A NEW CHOICE*
•*KNOW YOUR ENEMY* •*ENJOYING THE REMINDERS*

*As you prepare for your imminent release from the alcohol trap, it's time to cement a positive, excited mindset.*

In Chapter 8 I talked about the all-too-common phenomenon of the convict who reoffends soon after being released from prison, because he's frightened by the unfamiliarity of life on the outside. If you happened to know an ex-con like that, who was struggling to believe that he could cope with life outside prison, wouldn't you want to take him under your wing and show him how much better life is when you're free?

You'd probably begin by listing all the wonderful things you can do at your leisure, when you want to do them, not when you're permitted to do them. Things like:

• Seeing friends
• Going for a walk
• Driving a car
• Having a nice meal

- Going to the movies
- Sleeping late

Of course, he would know all these things, but he might have lost sight of just how enjoyable they are. When you're in prison and denied the usual pleasures in life, your idea of pleasure changes.

The alcohol trap is a prison. When you're addicted to alcohol, you lose the ability to enjoy the things you enjoyed before you started drinking. The alcohol-induced illusion of pleasure takes the place of genuine pleasures and becomes your be all and end all. But that's all it is: an illusion. The genuine pleasures still exist and they're still enjoyable. If you knew an ex-con who was struggling to see this and risking his freedom as a result, wouldn't you do everything in your power to make him see things as they really are?

If you could do that for someone else, why not do it for yourself? Think about all the pleasures that you have enjoyed in your life without drinking and start looking forward to enjoying those pleasures to the full again. It will help if you write them down. Your list may have a similar look to the example I gave for the ex-con, and the more you think about it, the more you will add to it. Take your time. There's no rush. What's important is that you establish the right frame of mind to quit with a feeling of excitement and certainty.

In Chapter 1 I explained how Easyway works like the combination to open a safe. In order to use the combination successfully you need to know all the numbers and apply them in the correct order. You may have found that frustrating at the time. You were eager to discover the cure to your drinking problem, and the prospect of reading through the whole book may have seemed laborious. But you have followed the instructions and now stand on the brink of becoming a happy nondrinker. You have come a long way toward achieving the state of mind necessary for you to quit and remain free for the rest of your life.

Congratulate yourself on your achievements. Remind yourself that there is no need to feel miserable; on the contrary, you have every reason to feel excited. You're setting yourself free from a prison that has brought you nothing but misery and stress and you're choosing a life that will bring you a happiness you may have forgotten even existed.

Perhaps you think that's an exaggeration and that you have no reason to congratulate yourself. You may be still feeling the effects of your drinking and struggling to convince yourself that this is going to be as easy as I say. It's time to address the fear of success.

## SEEING THINGS AS THEY REALLY ARE

The fear of life outside jail can keep the prisoner in the trap. He feels secure in his prison because it's an environment he knows. Even though it's a life of slavery, he fears it less than the world outside, which is alien and riddled with uncertainty.

When we relate this fear to stopping drinking, we have established that it's caused by illusions. These illusions have been put in your brain by many influences, each of which has a vested interest in you continuing to drink. You've been brainwashed into believing that drinking gives you some sort of pleasure or support.

You're also afraid that the process of stopping will be an ordeal that you will not be able to bear for long enough to succeed. Remember, with Easyway you succeed in becoming a nondrinker the moment you finish your final drink and feel no desire ever to drink again.

Some people see the alcohol trap as a hole in the ground: something you fall into easily but struggle to get out of. But that's not the case. Though it may feel like a deep, dark hole, there's no physical effort required to escape. You simply need to make a choice. It's a simple choice between taking a step backward or a step forward. You can either choose to remain in the trap for the rest of your life, becoming more and more enslaved and miserable, or you can choose the opposite:

### *FREEDOM*

There is no benefit whatsoever to being in the alcohol trap. You were lured into it by a set of illusions that were conjured up for you by people with a vested interest in you drinking. You took a step backward. And you've found that it makes you miserable. So now you just have to choose to do the opposite. Take a step forward. It's as simple as that. The fear of success can only stop you if you continue to believe that you get some pleasure or support from drinking.

Some of our fears are instinctive. For example, the fear of heights, fire, or the sea are natural responses that protect us from falling, getting burned, or drowning. There's nothing instinctive about the fear of escaping from the alcohol trap.

### *THE FEAR OF STOPPING DRINKING IS CREATED BY ALCOHOL ITSELF*

## IT'S YOUR DECISION

Once you're free from the alcohol trap, you'll be amazed at how easy it was to escape. You'll find that you're able to derive far more pleasure from life and your only regret will be not having made your escape sooner. At the moment you may still feel like someone struggling to get out of a deep pit, but once you do get out you'll realize your fears were groundless.

In order to achieve this success you need to clear your mind of all doubt. Understand and accept that your fears of trying to live without alcohol are based on illusions. In reality, you have nothing to fear.

On the subject of falling back into the trap, I'm sometimes asked, "How can you know for certain that something will not happen?" In other words, even if you do manage to quit drinking, how do you know you won't fall into the trap again? After all, the chances of being struck by a meteorite are infinitesimally small, yet nobody can say with absolute certainty that it will never happen to them.

That's very true; however, you have a considerable advantage over potential meteorite victims: If a meteorite is going to hit you, there's nothing you can do about it, whereas only you can make yourself go back to drinking. You control that decision and once you've seen through the confidence trick that lured you into the trap in the first place, you will have no difficulty in deciding to stay free.

If you still have doubts and fears at this stage, don't worry, that's not at all unusual. You've been brainwashed into thinking you have to go through some painful ordeal and make huge sacrifices to become a nondrinker, and that even if you do succeed, you will be forever tempted to drink again. I have explained that this is not the case and that recognizing this fact is purely a matter of changing the way you look at the situation. Once you're in the right frame of mind, you will change your perception and the fear will go.

My second instruction was to keep an open mind. If you have followed this instruction, you will have seen through the illusions to the true picture: that alcohol does absolutely nothing for you whatsoever. It's neither a source of pleasure nor support; in fact, it takes away genuine pleasures and leaves you feeling insecure. If you are still unclear on this point, go back and read through the book again, making sure you allow your mind to take it all on board.

Relax, let go of your preconceptions, and allow the true picture to take shape in your mind, like the STOP diagram in Chapter 6. The key to seeing through any illusion is not through willpower; it's through letting go of your existing perceptions and allowing your mind to see it another way.

## *ONCE YOU SEE THINGS AS THEY REALLY ARE, YOU CAN NEVER BE DELUDED AGAIN*

### NO GET-OUT CLAUSE

Some drinkers, once they get it into their head that it's just fear that prevents them from stopping, try to allay that fear by telling themselves they can always start again if it gets too hard—that quitting doesn't have to be final.

If you start off with that attitude, you're very likely to fail sooner or later, because you have allowed doubts to remain in your mind.

Instead, start off with the clear certainty that you're going to be free forever. Don't allow fear to continue to dictate your life.

## STEP FORWARD

You've already come a long way in the process of unraveling the brainwashing that has kept you hooked on alcohol and putting yourself in the right frame of mind to escape. Now you're going to start taking the practical forward steps that will see you become a happy nondrinker for the rest of your life.

Your first positive step was choosing to read this book. You had a choice: You could have continued to bury your head in the sand and stumble further and further into the miserable slavery of drinking.

Instead you decided to take positive action in order to resolve the situation. All I ask is that you continue making positive choices.

As we move forward, there are three very important facts that I want you to remember:

1. Alcohol does absolutely nothing for you at all.

It's crucial that you understand why this is so and accept it to be the case, so that you never get a feeling of deprivation or sacrifice.

2. There is no need for a transitional period.

With drug addicts this is often referred to as the "withdrawal period." But anyone who quits with Easyway has no need to worry about the withdrawal period. Yes, it may take time to repair the physical damage caused by alcohol, but the moment you stop drinking is the moment you become free. You don't have to wait for anything to happen.

3. There is no such thing as "just the one."

Just one drink is enough to make you a drinker and must be seen for what it is: part of a lifelong chain of self-destruction. People who see that there is no benefit to drinking alcohol have no desire to do so, not even "just the one."

## YOUR MORTAL ENEMY

Many addicts suffer the illusion that they can never get completely free. They convince themselves that their addiction is their friend, their confidence, their support, even part of their identity. They fear that if they quit they will not only lose their closest companion, they will lose a part of themselves.

It's a stark indication of just how severely the brainwashing distorts our perceptions, that anyone should come to regard something that is destroying them and making them miserable as a friend. When you lose a friend, you grieve. Eventually you come to terms with the loss and life goes on, but you may be left with a genuine void in your life that you can never fill. There's nothing you can do about it. You have no choice but to accept the situation and, though it still hurts, you do.

When drinkers, gamblers, smokers, heroin users, and other addicts try to quit by willpower, they feel they're losing a friend. They know that they're making the right decision to stop, but they still suffer a feeling of sacrifice and, therefore, there's a void in their lives. It isn't a genuine void, but they believe it is and so the effect is the same. They feel as if they're mourning for a friend. Yet this false friend isn't even dead. The purveyors of these drugs make absolutely sure that their victims are forever subjected to the temptation of forbidden fruit for the rest of their lives.

However, when you rid yourself of your mortal enemy, there is no need to mourn. On the contrary, you can rejoice and celebrate from the start, and you can continue to rejoice and celebrate for the rest of your life. Get it clear in your mind that alcohol is not your friend, nor is it part of your identity. It never has been. In fact, it's your mortal enemy and by getting rid of it you're sacrificing nothing, just making wonderful, positive gains.

So the answer to the question, "When will I be free?" is, "Whenever you choose to be." You could spend the next few days, and possibly the rest of your life, continuing to believe alcohol was your friend and wondering when you'll stop missing it. If so, you'll feel miserable, the desire to drink may never leave you, and you'll either end up feeling deprived for the rest of your life, or you'll end up going back to drinking and feeling even worse.

Alternatively, you can recognize alcohol for the mortal enemy that it really is and take pleasure in cutting it out of your life. Then you need never crave it again and whenever it enters your mind you'll feel elated that it's no longer destroying you.

Unlike people who quit with the willpower method, you'll be happy to think about your old enemy and you needn't try to block it from your mind. On the contrary, enjoy thinking about it and rejoice that it no longer plagues your life.

### DON'T MENTION THE ELEPHANT!

It's important that you don't try not to think about drinking after you've quit. Trying not to think about something is a sure way of becoming obsessed with it. If I tell you not to think about elephants, what's the first thing that comes into your head?

Exactly!

It's what you're thinking that's important. If you're thinking, "I'd love a drink, but I can't have one," you'll be miserable. But if you're thinking, "Isn't it wonderful, I don't have to drink any more, I'm free!" then you can think about drinking all you like and you'll be happy.

## REALIGN YOUR BRAIN

I asked you to approach this process with a relaxed, rational, and open mind, because that helps you understand the alcohol trap and the Little Monster that complains when you don't satisfy your urge to drink. During the first few days after your final drink, the Little Monster may be grumbling away, sending messages to your brain that it wants you to interpret as, "I want a drink."

But you now understand the true picture and, instead of drinking, or getting into a panic because you can't, pause for a moment. Take a deep breath. Remind yourself there is nothing to fear. There is no pain. The feeling isn't bad. It's just the slight uncomfortable feeling that occurs when alcohol leaves your system. It's what drinkers suffer throughout their drinking lives.

In the past your mind interpreted the pangs of the Little Monster as "I want a drink" because it had every reason to believe that alcohol would satisfy the empty, insecure feeling. But now you understand that, far from relieving that feeling, it's alcohol that caused it.

So just relax, accept the feeling for what it really is— the death throes of the Little Monster—and remind yourself, "Nondrinkers don't have this problem. This is a feeling that drinkers suffer and they suffer it throughout their drinking lives. Isn't it great! It will soon be gone forever."

## THE WITHDRAWAL PANGS WILL CEASE TO FEEL LIKE PANGS AND WILL BECOME MOMENTS OF PLEASURE

During the first few days in particular you might well find that you forget you've quit. It can happen at any time. You think, "I'll have a drink," and then you remember with joy that you're now a nondrinker. But you wonder why the thought entered your head when you were convinced you'd reversed the brainwashing. Such times can be crucial in whether you succeed or not. React in the wrong way and they can be disastrous. Doubts can surface and you may start to question your decision to quit and lose faith in yourself.

These occurrences won't catch you out if you're prepared for them. Have your mindset ready so that when they occur you remain calm and use them as a reminder of the wonderful freedom you've gained. Instead of thinking, "I can't do this," you will think, "Isn't it great! I don't need to drink anymore. I'm free!"

The associations that you had with drinking, such as seeing friends, eating out, going to parties, etc, can linger on after the Little Monster has died. For drinkers who quit with the willpower method, this can seriously undermine their efforts. In their minds they have built up a powerful case against drinking, they've decided to become a nondrinker, they've managed to go for however long without drinking, and yet on certain occasions a voice keeps saying, "I want a drink." They haven't killed the Big Monster and so they still think of drinking as a pleasure or support.

Although you will no longer suffer the illusion that you're being deprived, it's still imperative that you prepare yourself for these situations.

Occasionally forgetting that you no longer drink isn't a bad sign; it's a very good one. It's proof that your life is returning to the happy state you were in before you got hooked on alcohol, when your whole existence wasn't dominated by a poisonous and highly addictive drug.

Expecting these moments to happen and being prepared for them means you won't be caught off guard. You'll be wearing a suit of impregnable armor. You know you've made the correct decision and nobody will be able to make you doubt it. Instead of being the cause of your downfall, these moments will give you added strength, security, and pleasure, reminding you just how wonderful it is to be

*FREE!*

## SUMMARY

- Addiction is not a hole in the ground—there is no physical effort required to get out.

- It's easy to get out of the alcohol trap—you just have to make a different choice.

- Have no doubts about the choice you're making and be certain that you will succeed.

- Remember, alcohol does nothing for you whatsoever.

- There's nothing to wait for. The moment you stop drinking is the moment you become free.

- There's no such thing as "just one drink." If you take one drink, you will take another and another and be back in the trap.

- Rejoice at ridding yourself of your mortal enemy.

# Chapter 14

# TAKING CONTROL

**IN THIS CHAPTER**

• *WHO PULLS THE STRINGS?* • *THE MYTH OF CHOICE*

• *RECOGNIZING YOU HOLD THE KEY AND USING IT*

• *OWNING UP* • *THE THRILL OF GETTING YOUR LIFE BACK*

*Problem drinkers are tormented by their inability to control their drinking. You regain control as soon as you start to make choices based on facts rather than illusions.*

The brainwashing can only fool you to a certain extent. Despite the abundance of misinformation designed to keep us in the alcohol trap, all drinkers are acutely aware of the many good reasons not to drink. The frequent attempts to stop or cut down are driven by one or more of these reasons, but it's only when you succeed in stopping that you realize the greatest gain to be had from quitting: to escape from slavery.

Drinkers hate the thought that they have become slaves. Like Rachel on page 116, a lot of problem drinkers are very strong-willed people who have enjoyed a high degree of control over most of their lives and it frustrates them to think that they're being controlled by something they despise. They think they should be able to conquer their problem through sheer force of will and the fact that they can't leaves them feeling depressed and frustrated.

The reason they can't quit through willpower is because they're caught in a trap that they don't understand. Just like pushing on the hinged side of a door, they find themselves frustrated because they're going about it the wrong way. They assume that if all the terrible things they know about alcohol aren't enough to make them stop, there must be something wrong with them. But they're missing the point.

## WE DON'T DRINK FOR THE REASONS WE SHOULDN'T, WE DRINK FOR THE REASONS WE DO

In reality, these "reasons" are all illusions. However, until they are removed, focusing on why we shouldn't drink is counterproductive. The tragedy of the willpower method is that even if you do succeed in stopping you still do not attain freedom. You waste your life moping for something that you pray you're not going to have! That's an absurd and intolerable situation to put yourself in. You can't win!

The thing that really makes drinkers miserable is not so much the threat of liver failure, or even destroying their relationships, or throwing their money down the drain; it's the feeling of powerlessness to quit doing something that they know is ruining their lives. It's:

### THE SHEER SLAVERY

Such is their desperation that they search for any flimsy excuse to keep drinking and they block out the people who are trying to help them. They try to close their minds to the terrible effects of being a drinker. But these lurk like dark shadows at the back of their mind and the deeper they descend into the pit, the darker the shadows become.

Health is the most common reason drinkers give for wanting to quit. Perhaps they start to feel an ache around the kidneys, or they can't sleep, or they keep getting headaches. There are countless alcohol-induced ailments that set the alarm bells ringing.

Money is another common reason given for quitting. Pouring thousands of pounds down the drain that they can't afford leads to severe stress, and it's not unusual for a problem drinker to squander more than $400,000 in a lifetime on alcohol.

The social effects of drinking are also a reason for wanting to quit. The effect that alcohol has on your moods and behavior, and how that affects family and friends, can be devastating. If you're fortunate enough to recognize it before it's too late, then the damage you're doing to your relationships and the pain you're causing people you care about can be reversed.

On the flip side, ask a drinker why they drink and they will nearly always react defensively and negatively. They can't seem to find good reasons why they do, but resort to excuses for why they haven't stopped.

"It's not killing me."

"I can take it or leave it."

"There are worse things I could do."

Is that the sign of a genuine pleasure? If you ask someone why they watch baseball, or go to the movies, or visit art galleries, or listen to music, do they say, "There are worse things I could do"? When something gives you genuine pleasure, you're only too anxious to enthuse about it. You don't make excuses for why you don't stop doing it!

Defensiveness is a sure sign of someone who knows they're not in control and feels trapped. The key that enables addicts to get free is the realization that they have the power to walk out of the trap: They no longer need to be a slave to drinking; they won't miss drinking; they will enjoy life more; they will be able to deal better with stress; they won't have to go through some terrible ordeal in order to escape.

When you succeed in stopping, you will look back on your days as a drinker and rejoice in your newfound freedom—the freedom to look at other drinkers, not with envy or deprivation, but with pity, just as you would look upon a heroin addict. The greatest gain to be made from becoming a nondrinker is not so much the good health, the money or the social stability—although they're fantastic bonuses—but to no longer feel like a pathetic, helpless slave.

## WHAT'S YOUR POISON?

I'm sure you have a favorite drink? One of the ingenious illusions of the alcohol trap, and one that is relentlessly pushed by the people who market alcoholic drinks, is that drinkers should be discerning in their choice of poison. The most obvious example is wine, an industry that has woven an elaborate mesh of snobbery around its product—fermented grape juice—to the extent that wine connoisseurs will gather and talk nonsense for hours on end about grape varieties, soil structures, climate, etc.

And the wine industry is not alone. A similar mystique has long existed around spirits, particularly single malt whisky, with its characteristic flavors of peat and brine. Can you think of anything more disgusting than swallowing earth or sea water! And these days we're even expected to look for the subtle nuances in beer!

This image of "the discerning connoisseur" is a very clever ruse designed to keep you in the trap by deluding you into thinking you're in control. You're not just throwing any old addictive poison down your throat; you're making an educated choice.

### WISE UP!

In reality, the only choice that matters is whether you drink or don't drink.

Funnily enough, when it comes to this decision, drinkers become aware that they're not, in fact, in control. They're very familiar with all the powerful reasons to not drink, yet they feel powerless to resist the urge.

When you first start drinking, the illusion of control is very strong. As you slide further into the trap, your tolerance to the drug increases, and so you require more to relieve the craving. You start to drink more and more often. You still believe you're in control but if you tried to stop you would feel some hidden power preventing you.

Now you're drinking to the extent that you know it will have an impact on your way of life. Like a bad dream, you're watching yourself turn into an alcoholic—something you thought only happened to other people—and you're helpless to do anything about it.

You're becoming incapable of meeting your responsibilities and fulfilling simple tasks. You're becoming forgetful and irritable. You try to hide your problem by lying to those closest to you. You sense that you're putting everything you value in jeopardy, yet you feel powerless.

This conflict creates a feeling of self-loathing, which often expresses itself as irritability towards others. When you're in the alcohol trap, you're pulled in opposite directions. Part of your brain is telling you not to drink, but another part is compelling you to keep drinking. It leaves you in a constant state of confusion: If you want to stop, why can't you just do so? With other things in life, if you wanted to stop and had very good reasons to do so, you would, so why can't you apply the same control with drinking?

The answer is simple:

### *WHEN YOU DRINK, YOU'RE NOT IN CONTROL*

There is a force controlling you, compelling you to make choices that go against your instincts. That force has a name: addiction.

## A CHOICE BASED ON ILLUSIONS

Who makes you drink? Has anyone ever held a gun to your head and said, "Drink!"? Every time you bring the bottle or glass to your lips, you're taking the conscious decision to drink. You may think that contradicts my previous statement that you're not in control. In fact it doesn't. Your addiction to alcohol is making you take that decision.

### *YOU DON'T CONTROL ALCOHOL, ALCOHOL CONTROLS YOU*

Like the fly in the pitcher plant, we're controlled from the moment we're drawn to our first drink. As we descend into the pit, we become increasingly torn between the desire to cut down or stop and the desire to increase our intake.

This constant battle goes on in every addict's mind. It's confusing and makes us feel foolish and powerless. Nobody likes to feel that way, so we go into denial; we bury our head in the sand in order to avoid facing the painful truth about what we've become: a hopeless, pathetic slave to alcohol. Instead of facing up to this unpleasant reality and confronting our fears, we carry on making excuses for continuing to drink.

As long as you go on conning yourself that you're in control of your drinking, you will fail to do the one thing that will solve your problem: quit. Only when you understand and accept that alcohol controls you, not the other way round, can you see that the only way to regain control of your life is to stop.

Not only is it the only way, it's the easy way. Go on insisting that you're in control and you will remain a slave.

Do you see now how willpower keeps you in the trap? On the willpower method, you continue to believe that you're giving up a genuine pleasure or crutch so you sentence yourself to a lifetime of hardship. Let go of that illusion and escape will be easy.

The alcohol trap is an ingenious prison, but it has one fatal flaw. The prisoners hold the key to their own release. In order for them to escape, three things must happen:

1.  They must recognize that they're in a trap.

2.  They must recognize that they hold the key.

3.  They must be shown how to use the key.

Easyway is the only method that does this. Everything I have told you so far was designed to help you see the trap that you're in and recognize that you hold the key. The trap is the addiction. The key is unraveling the brainwashing that keeps you addicted—killing the Big Monster. The final step is to turn the key—to kill the Little Monster – and walk free.

I have explained about the alcohol trap and how it keeps you hooked by creating the illusion of pleasure. By now you should be completely clear that any benefit you thought you got from alcohol was merely an illusion created by a combination of the Little and Big Monsters. You should be in no doubt that alcohol provides neither pleasure nor support. It does not give you courage. It does not make you more interesting or entertaining, nor does it help you to be calm. It's not a reward, it's pure punishment—a highly addictive poison that destroys you physically and mentally. If you have any lingering doubts about any of these points, I urge you to go back and read through from Chapter 5. It's essential that you kill the Big Monster before you make your final escape.

You should also be clear that the only way to control alcohol is not to drink. Cutting down or just having "the odd one" is not the best of both worlds; it's the worst of both worlds. As long as you put alcohol in your system, alcohol will control you. The only people who are not controlled by alcohol are nondrinkers. You become a nondrinker the moment you stop drinking without any desire ever to drink again.

From that moment the Little Monster will begin to die. This is nothing to fear. On the contrary, you should rejoice in its death throes. Remember, it's your mortal enemy and it's leaving you for good. The fear that has prevented you from escaping from the drinking trap before now is the fear that you won't be able to enjoy or cope with life without drinking. Nondrinkers don't have this fear. Drinking doesn't relieve it; it causes it. It's fantastic to be free of this fear.

## CONFESSION

A major cause of stress for drinkers is the effort they go to to keep their problem secret. It's much easier to overcome any problem if you're open and honest about it. But perhaps you find the idea of owning up unthinkable. You're afraid that people will be angry and will lose respect for you. I admit it's possible that this will be the case. The people who love and trust you will be hurt, but in the end they will respect you for coming clean and will want to help.

It's more than likely that the people you think you've been deceiving haven't been deceived at all. They will have noticed the change in your behavior. They will already have been hurt by your irritability. They will have become suspicious of your inability to apply yourself to work and other commitments. The longer you go on trying to deceive them, the more these feelings will grow into distrust and alienation. Come clean and you give them the opportunity to understand why your behavior has changed and to help you sort it out. Don't be surprised to find that they're relieved by your admission.

You may feel that your loved ones are not ready for the full story of your alcohol addiction and that "dumping it on them" would be unfair. That's fine. You're the best person to judge when the time is right to share the truth. Once you're enjoying the confidence and self-respect that comes with your newfound freedom, you will be better equipped to work out the best way to come clean.

## ENJOY BREAKING FREE

When you find that you're enjoying life and coping with stress better as a nondrinker, you will no longer have to try to block your mind to the terrible effects that drinking had on you both physically and mentally. One of the huge bonuses of quitting is that you will no longer need to worry about them.

It's time to kill the Little Monster and make your escape from the alcohol trap. Remember, fear is not relieved by drinking; it is caused by it. You have nothing to fear from stopping, only wonderful gains to make. Think about the fly on the funnel of the pitcher plant. You could set it free by encouraging it to fly out while it still has a chance.

See yourself as a nondrinker sees you. Remember, alcohol does absolutely nothing for you whatsoever. It's a poison that causes immense damage to the length and quality of your life. You can stop the damage immediately by never drinking again. You have nothing to lose and everything to gain.

What do you think when you see a heroin addict? Isn't it obvious that each time they inject the drug into a vein they're not curing their problem but making it worse and that the only thing that will end the problem for them is to stop taking heroin?

Think about the ex-con who's in danger of jeopardizing his freedom by reoffending, because he's afraid of life outside prison. Put yourself in his position. Remind him of all the wonderful advantages there are to being free. Remind yourself of all the wonderful gains you will make without alcohol in your life.

• Better health

- Fewer mood swings
- Better relationships
- Higher self-esteem
- Less stress
- Better sleep
- Better concentration
- Clearer thinking
- More money

### AND MOST IMPORTANT OF ALL

- Control over your life

This is your chance to fly free. In fact, you can fly free any time you choose, so why wait? You have nothing to fear. Remember, dreadful things are guaranteed to happen as long as you stay in the alcohol trap.

Escape and you can take control of putting your life back together. You will be amazed by how good it feels to be free from the slavery of drinking.

Very soon I'm going to ask you to make a solemn vow that you will never drink alcohol again. First, there is one final stage that we need to prepare for. It's called withdrawal.

## SUMMARY

- Stop being a slave to alcohol.
- The addiction controls you.
- The only way to control alcohol is to stop drinking.
- Free yourself and you will be amazed how good life feels.

Chapter 15

# WITHDRAWAL

## IN THIS CHAPTER

•*FEAR OF THE PAIN*  •*THAT PANIC FEELING*
•*WITHDRAWAL SYMPTOMS*  •*KILLING THE LITTLE MONSTER*
•*WHEN DOES IT END?*  •*PREPARING FOR YOUR FINAL DRINK*

*When you quit with Easyway, any withdrawal symptoms become a source of pleasure, not pain.*

Throughout the book I have talked about withdrawal as the feeling that we interpret as "I want a drink"—the Little Monster that cries out for alcohol. I have explained that this feeling is so slight as to be almost imperceptible. Perhaps you've assumed that I'm talking about a different withdrawal from the one you go through when you quit for good.

There is a common misconception among drinkers that in order to stop drinking permanently you have to endure a painful withdrawal period as all the toxins leave your body. You will have heard of delirium tremens—the DTs—and other feverish symptoms that afflict withdrawing alcoholics. The fear of these symptoms is enough to prevent a lot of drinkers from even trying to quit. As with all the other reasons drinkers give for not stopping, it's a myth.

Most drinkers who quit experience no abnormal physical symptoms during withdrawal, no sweats or shakes, no headaches or palpitations. We only think we have to go through some terrible trauma because stopping on the willpower method can be psychological torture and that can itself create physical symptoms. But every night, millions of drinkers manage to sleep for eight hours and when they wake up they're not in agony after having to go so long without their drug. If the physical effects of withdrawal were so bad, it would wake them up during the night, desperate for a drink. But most drinkers manage to last well into the day before they have their first drink. Not only are they getting by quite happily without any physical pain, they're not even aware of any discomfort.

Sure, they probably look forward to their first drink and if someone stood in their way and prevented them from having it they might well get very angry, but that is not a reaction to physical pain; that's panic at the thought of being deprived. When you're confident of having your next drink, this panic recedes. If it were a physical pain, it would be there all the time, like toothache.

## AVOIDING PANIC

Most problem drinkers are familiar with the "panic feeling" that sets in when they don't know where the next drink is coming from. It's like a smoker running out of cigarettes. Smokers will go to great lengths to replenish their supply, often walking miles through the rain, late at night just to stock up on their little "crutch." Drinkers too will make incredible efforts to ensure they're not denied the opportunity to drink, sneaking out of the house, lying about where they're going, and even putting themselves in dangerous situations.

But occasionally you meet a heavy drinker who claims not to know the panic feeling. We know that drinkers lie, to others and to themselves, but there are some who genuinely never feel this panic of not knowing where their next drink is going to come from, for the simple reason that they're so frightened of finding themselves in that position that they take every precaution to make sure it never happens! In other words, far from being less affected by the panic than most drinkers, they're even more consumed by it.

The truth is that every drinker who is denied the opportunity to drink when they expect to experiences the panic feeling. But this is not the same as physical pain, and when you remove the desire to drink, the panic disappears.

## WITHDRAWAL SYMPTOMS

So let's examine just how serious withdrawal can get. You may have read about the symptoms:

- Anxiety
- Irritability
- Mood swings
- Nervousness
- Depression
- Confusion

First, these are not physical symptoms, they're psychological. Second, they're symptoms that every drinker suffers to a greater or lesser degree, WHILE THEY'RE DRINKING. These symptoms are all caused by alcohol, so the one way to guarantee that you suffer them is to go on drinking.

The physical symptoms you may have seen mentioned include:

- Tiredness
- Headaches
- Stomach upsets
- Weak and aching muscles
- Heart palpitations
- The shakes
- The sweats
- The shivers
- Difficult breathing

This set of symptoms is very similar to the symptoms of flu; in fact, they're often described as such. No doubt you've had flu on several occasions in your life and you probably expect to get it again, but the thought of getting flu doesn't induce panic. Even though flu can make us feel lousy, we can put up with it relatively easily.

If I offered you a deal: a week's flu in exchange for a lifetime of freedom and happiness, wouldn't you take it?

Even if the withdrawal symptoms were painful, wouldn't you endure a little pain in exchange for your freedom from slavery to alcohol?

The fact is we're very well equipped to endure pain. Just as an experiment, try squeezing your thigh and digging your fingernails in, gradually increasing the pressure.

You'll find you can endure quite a severe level of pain without any fear or panic. That's because you're in control. You know what's causing the pain and you know that you can make it stop whenever you choose.

Now repeat the exercise and when the pain is as much as you can bear, try to imagine that it wasn't you causing it but that it had just suddenly started and that you knew neither the cause nor how long it would last. Now imagine that pain being in your head or chest. You would immediately panic.

Pain is not the problem; the problem is the fear and panic that pain induces if you don't understand why you're feeling it or what the consequences might be.

In fact, we often panic at the slightest feeling of discomfort if we don't know what's caused it and fear it might be the beginning of something severe.

Observe drinkers, especially when they're denied the opportunity to drink. They'll be restless and fidgety. You'll notice little nervous tics, they'll be constantly doing things with their hands or grinding their teeth. This restlessness is triggered by an empty, insecure feeling, which can quickly turn into frustration, irritability, anxiety, anger, fear, and panic if they're not able to satisfy their alcohol craving.

Get it clear in your mind: Alcohol causes this feeling, it doesn't relieve it. As long as you understand that, you don't need to feel any sense of deprivation when you stop.

## *IF YOU CONTINUE TO DRINK, YOU'LL SUFFER THAT EMPTY, INSECURE FEELING FOR THE REST OF YOUR LIFE*

## A WILLFUL AGONY

The psychological symptoms I listed on page 194 are what drinkers suffer when they try to quit with the willpower method. Perhaps you've experienced this yourself. They're all symptoms of anxiety, induced by the feeling that they're being deprived of their pleasure or support. As long as you believe that you're being deprived, the almost imperceptible withdrawal pangs—the tiny cries of the Little Monster—will continue to induce fear and panic and you may suffer physically.

Ignorance and illusion are the twin evils that combine to turn a small signal in your brain into panic and mental torture. Imagine having a permanent itch that you were not allowed to scratch. Imagine how that would torment you and think about the amount of willpower you would have to summon up to resist scratching the itch just once. Imagine also that you believed the itch would last for the rest of your life unless you were allowed to scratch it.

How long do you think you could last before you scratched the itch? If you did manage to hold out for a week or even more, imagine the relief you would feel when you finally gave in.

This is a description of the torture that drinkers go through when trying to quit with the willpower method. For them the urge to scratch the itch lasts long after the Little Monster has died. It's triggered by everything they ever associated with drinking, such as unwinding after a day's work, meeting friends, and going to parties. They think, "I used to drink on these occasions," and they still believe they're being deprived. The Big Monster is still alive, telling them that they need to scratch the itch.

Remember, the perception of drinking as a pleasure or support is a figment of your imagination, left over from the brainwashing. It's like applying an ointment to a spot in the belief that it will clear it up, when all it does is turn the spot into a rash. If you were in that situation and I told you all you had to do was leave the spot for a few days and it would clear up on its own, you would have no need or desire for the ointment.

When you have your final drink, you will find it easy to become a nondrinker because you will realize that the empty, insecure feeling of wanting a drink was caused by the last drink you had, and that the one thing that would insure you suffer that feeling for the rest of your life would be to drink another. You will experience none of the suffering that you went through on previous attempts because you will no longer believe you are being deprived. On the contrary, you'll experience a wonderful feeling of freedom. Once you realize that the pleasure or support is just an illusion, you will feel no deprivation and, consequently, no misery or torture. Just a wonderful feeling of elation.

## THE PLEASURE OF WITHDRAWAL

When you've finished your final drink, you may be aware of the withdrawal for a few days. Remember, this is not a physical pain, it's just the faint cries of the Little Monster wanting to be fed. However, light though it is, you should not ignore it.

It's essential to keep in mind the fact that the Little Monster was created when you first started drinking and it has continued to feed on every subsequent drink you've had. As soon as you stop drinking, you cut off the supply and it begins to die.

In its death throes the Little Monster will try to entice you to feed it. Create a mental image of this parasite getting weaker and weaker and enjoy starving it to death. Keep this mental image with you at all times and make sure you don't respond to its death throes by thinking, "I need a drink."

Remember that the empty, insecure feeling was caused by your last drink. The feeling itself isn't pleasurable, but you will enjoy it because you will understand the cause and know that the Little Monster inside you is dying.

It's like vigorous exercise. When you push yourself hard it becomes uncomfortable, but the feeling doesn't make you panic. You enjoy the feeling because you know that you control it and that it's an indication that you're doing yourself good.

Take a sadistic delight in killing off the Little Monster. Even if you do get that feeling of "I want a drink" for a few days, don't worry about it. Remember, it's not a drink you want; it's relief from that nagging feeling which will go away permanently provided you never drink again. If you were to have a drink, it would guarantee you suffer it for the rest of your life. It's just the Little Monster doing everything it can to tempt you to feed it. As long as you see that, you will find it easy to starve it to death. You now have complete control over it. It's no longer destroying you; you're destroying it and soon you will be free forever.

## WHEN CAN I RELAX?

You're probably thinking, "OK, but how long before I'm cured?" The good news is you can start enjoying the genuine pleasure of being a nondrinker from the moment you finish your final drink. Unlike the willpower method, with Easyway you don't have to wait for anything.

It takes just a few days for the physical withdrawal to pass. During this time, people who use the willpower method tend to feel completely obsessed with being denied what they see as their pleasure or support. Then, after about three weeks, there may come a moment when they suddenly realize that they have not thought about drinking for a while. It's an exciting feeling... and a dangerous moment.

They've gone from believing that life will always be miserable without being able to drink, to believing that time will solve their problem. They feel great—surely this is the cure. It's time to celebrate. What possible harm could it do to reward themselves with just one drink?

Clearly the Big Monster is still alive. They still believe that they have been denying themselves some sort of pleasure. If they're stupid enough to have a drink, they won't find it rewarding at all. It will give them no feeling of pleasure or support. The only reason they ever experienced the illusion of pleasure from drinking is that it partially relieved the symptoms of withdrawal. But now that they're no longer withdrawing from alcohol, they will not even experience that illusion.

But that one drink is enough to revive the Little Monster. Now panic starts to creep back in. They don't want their efforts to quit to be blown away so easily and for nothing, so they draw on their willpower and try not to give in to the urge to drink again. But after a while the same thing happens. They regain their confidence and the temptation to have "just the one" rears its ugly head again. This time they can say to themselves, "I did it last time and didn't get hooked, so what's the harm in doing it again?" They're wandering back into the trap.

Does this ring any bells? Anyone who has tried to quit with the willpower method is likely to have experienced something similar. With Easyway, when you realize you haven't thought about drinking for a while, your first thought is not to celebrate with a drink, it's

### YIPPEE! I'M FREE!

There is no feeling of deprivation. You can relax from the moment you finish your final drink, and rather than interpreting the feeling as "I want a drink", you think, "Yippee! Isn't it wonderful! I don't ever have to go through that misery again."

Many ex-drinkers who quit with the willpower method never get to the point where they can say that with certainty. They're never quite sure whether they've kicked it. The physical withdrawal symptoms feel like normal anxiety and stress, so when they experience these feelings they interpret them as "I want a drink." Of course, drinking at this stage wouldn't even give the illusion of relieving these natural pangs as they have no withdrawal, but they don't know that. They're still convinced that alcohol will help. The real stress is now increased because they believe that they're being deprived of a support that will ease the situation.

They're faced with a dilemma: Go through the rest of their life believing they're missing out, or find out for sure. Sadly, the only way to do that is to drink again. If they do, they find that their stress is not relieved—in fact, it's increased by their sense of disappointment at having giving in to temptation. But they've revived the Little Monster and the outcome is that pretty soon they'll be drinking just as before.

## THE MOMENT OF TRUTH

Soon you'll have your final drink and make a solemn vow never to drink again. If this thought makes you panic, remind yourself of these simple facts:

- The alcoholic drinks industry depends on that panic to keep you hooked.
- Alcohol doesn't relieve the panic; it causes it.

Take a moment to compose yourself. Do you really have any reason to panic? Nothing bad is going to happen as a result of you stopping drinking. You have only wonderful gains to make.

Perhaps you're afraid of going into unknown territory. There is nothing unknown about what you're about to do. It's something you've already done thousands of times before, every time you've drained your last glass at the end of the evening. This particular drink will be a very, very special one. It will be your last.

---

**ALREADY STOPPED?**

If you stopped drinking before you started reading this book, that's fine, provided you're confident that you have killed the Big Monster and you have no doubts whatsoever that you're not making a sacrifice or depriving yourself in any way. It's still important that you make the vow.

---

Very soon you will feel stronger, both physically and mentally. You will have more energy, more confidence, more self-respect, and more money. It's essential that you don't put off this wonderful freedom, not for a week, a day, or a second. Waiting for something to happen is one of the reasons why drinkers using the willpower method find it so difficult. What are they waiting for? To find out if they'll ever drink again? There's only one way to find that out... so instead they're just left waiting, waiting, for the rest of their lives.

You become a nondrinker the moment you finish your final drink. What you're achieving is a new frame of mind, an understanding that drinking does nothing for you and that by not drinking you're freeing yourself from a life of slavery, misery, and degradation.

Replace any panic you may have felt with a feeling of

excitement. You no longer need to be sick, incapable, secretive, or dishonest. You're about to discover the joy of taking control. Rejoice! This is going to be one of the best experiences you've ever had.

### *YOU'RE ABOUT TO BECOME FREE!*

---

## SUMMARY

- The ordeal of withdrawal is psychological, not physical, and Allen Carr's Easyway removes it.

- See the physical withdrawal as the death throes of the Little Monster and enjoy killing it off.

- Be aware that everyday pangs such as anxiety and stress feel the same as withdrawal, but drinking will not relieve them.

- Drinkers suffer withdrawal pangs all the time. Nondrinkers don't suffer them at all.

- Get into a positive frame of mind: Feel the excitement of what you're achieving.

# Chapter 16

# PREPARING TO QUIT

**IN THIS CHAPTER**
*•FINAL CHECKS*
*•CHOOSING YOUR MOMENT*
*•THE RIGHT TIME IS NOW*

*It's time for some final checks before you make your leap to freedom.*

Earlier I compared the feeling of freedom when you escape the alcohol trap to the exhilaration of a parachute jump. What you're about to do will be one of the most exciting experiences of your life, so let's make sure that everything goes to plan and run through a final checklist to make sure you're properly prepared.

### 1. FEEL EAGER AND EXCITED

Your frame of mind should be, "Great! I don't need to drink any more. I'm about to free myself from a prison of misery and degradation. I can't wait!"

You have every reason to celebrate. You're about to walk free from an evil trap, which has kept you imprisoned and severely disrupted your life, making you miserable, confused, frightened, and angry. You're about to regain control over your life and banish those feelings of slavery and powerlessness for good.

Very soon you will be a nondrinker. Take pride in your achievement; there are millions of drinkers in the world who wish they could be in your shoes. Soon you will rediscover the unbridled joy of feeling healthy, having nothing to hide, having time for the people you love and the things you love to do. While you were in the alcohol trap you forgot how to enjoy the genuine pleasures in life. You're about to get that huge part of your life back.

## 2. DISPEL THE ILLUSIONS

We have unraveled the brainwashing and dispelled the illusions that made you believe that drinking gave you pleasure and support. You know and understand that alcohol is an addictive poison that will eventually destroy you, physically and mentally. You have seen through the myths that kept you in the drinking trap. You know that alcohol doesn't relieve stress and anxiety, it causes them; it's not a social lubricant, it's a social saboteur; it doesn't give you courage, it undermines it; and it doesn't help you think, it impairs judgment.

## 3. SEE THE TRUE PICTURE

The reason you have not been able to stop drinking permanently before is not because there is something wonderful about alcohol that you can't live without, nor is it a flaw in your personality. It's because you followed the wrong method.

Now you understand that alcohol gives you neither pleasure nor support, and the only reason you ever thought it did was because each drink brought a little bit of relief from the craving caused by the drink before. You have been addicted to a drug that takes control away from you but still tricks you into thinking you're in control. You have accepted that alcohol made you a slave and the only way to escape that slavery is to stop.

### 4. REMOVE ALL DOUBT

If you can accept items 1, 2 and 3 above, you should also be able to accept item 4. As you prepare to take your final drink and quit drinking for good, you should be in no doubt that the decision you're taking isn't just the right one; it's the only one if you don't want to spend the rest of your life as a slave to alcohol.

You understand that any lingering pangs after you stop are just the cries of the Little Monster as it breathes its last. Enjoy the feeling—it's the feeling of freedom. Nothing can distract you now.

If you don't feel able to accept all four points, if you have doubts about what you're about to do, it means that you haven't understood something and you need to go back and re-read it until you do. Don't be downhearted. A lot of people get to this stage and feel unsure about something. It nearly always turns out to be just a small detail that they haven't quite grasped. All it takes is to go back and read it again, and you suddenly understand.

To help you identify any gaps you feel need filling, we've supplied a prompt at the end of this chapter. Take a look at the code word, RATIONALIZED, on page 212. Go through each item and ask yourself:

- Do I understand it?
- Do I agree with it?
- Am I following it?

If you have any doubts, reread the relevant chapters as listed.

Stopping with Easyway is not difficult. All you need to do is follow the instructions and you will succeed. If you're finding that hard to accept, it could be because you still believe you have to go through some sort of ordeal. Relax. Open your mind. Let go of all the misconceptions that kept you in the trap and allow your mind to embrace the truth.

If you have achieved the right frame of mind and your checklist is complete, you're fully equipped to succeed at something that most ex-drinkers regard as the most important and significant achievement of their life. If you feel like a dog straining at the leash, eager to get on with it, that's great. All I ask is that you finish the book.

## THE IDEAL MOMENT TO QUIT

Very soon you will undertake the ritual of your final drink. You may be wondering when would be the ideal moment? Let's look at your options.

There are two typical occasions that tend to trigger attempts to quit, whether it's drinking, smoking, gambling, or anything else that is disrupting your life. One is a traumatic event, such as a health scare or a financial blow, the other is a "special" day, such as a birthday or New Year's Day. I call these "meaningless days" because they actually have no bearing whatsoever on your drinking, other than providing a target date for you to make your attempt to stop. That would be fine if it helped, but meaningless days actually cause more harm than good.

New Year's Day is the most popular of all meaningless days, being a clear marker of the end of one period and the beginning of another. It also happens to have the lowest success rate. The Christmas holidays are a time when we drink more than usual and by New Year's Eve we're just about ready for a break.

So we have one last binge and then, as the clock strikes midnight, we vow that we'll give the stuff a miss. We very quickly start to feel cleansed, but the Little Monster is demanding its fix. If we're using the wrong method, we interpret these cries as "I want a drink," and though we may hold out to begin with, eventually the Big Monster will have its way and we find ourselves back in the trap.

Meaningless days only encourage us to go through the damaging cycle of halfhearted attempts to quit, bringing on the feeling of deprivation, followed by the sense of failure that reinforces the illusion that stopping is difficult and may be impossible. Drinkers spend their lives looking for excuses to put off "the dreaded day." Meaningless days provide the perfect excuse to say, "I will quit, just not today."

Then there are the days when something shakes your world

and you respond by saying it's time to sort yourself out. But these stressful times are also when your desire to drink becomes strongest, because you regard alcohol as a form of support. This is another ingenuity of the trap:

### *NO MATTER WHICH DAY YOU CHOOSE TO QUIT, IT ALWAYS SEEMS TO BE WRONG*

Some drinkers choose their annual vacation, thinking that they'll be able to cope better away from the everyday stresses of work and home life and the usual temptations to drink. Others pick a time when there are no social events coming up where they will find it difficult not to drink. These approaches might work for a while, but they leave a lingering doubt: "OK, I've coped so far, but what about when I go back to work or that big party comes around?"

When you quit with Easyway, we encourage you to go out and handle stress and throw yourself into social occasions right away, so that you can prove to yourself from the start that, even at times when you feared you would find it hard to cope without drinking, you're still happy to be free.

So what is the best time to quit?

If you saw someone you love hurting themselves repeatedly, what would you say? Would you ask them to stop the next time a convenient moment arises? Or would you ask them to stop at once?

## THE IDEAL MOMENT TO STOP IS NOW

That's what the people who love you would say if they knew about your drinking problem. You have everything you need to quit. Like an athlete on the blocks at the start of the race, you're in peak condition to insure success.

Think of everything you have to gain: a life free from slavery, dishonesty, misery, anger, deceit, self-loathing, impotence. No more scratching around for money; no more lying to people about what you need it for; no more hiding yourself away or trying to cover your tracks; no more feeling disappointed, guilty, and weak.

In place of all that misery you can look forward to living in the light, with your head held high, enjoying open, honest relationships with the people around you, feeling in control of how you spend your time and money, and finding joy in the genuine pleasures that you enjoyed before you walked into the alcohol trap.

With so much happiness to gain and so much misery to rid yourself of, what possible reason is there to wait? It's time for my sixth instruction:

### DON'T WAIT FOR THE RIGHT TIME TO QUIT

### DO IT NOW!

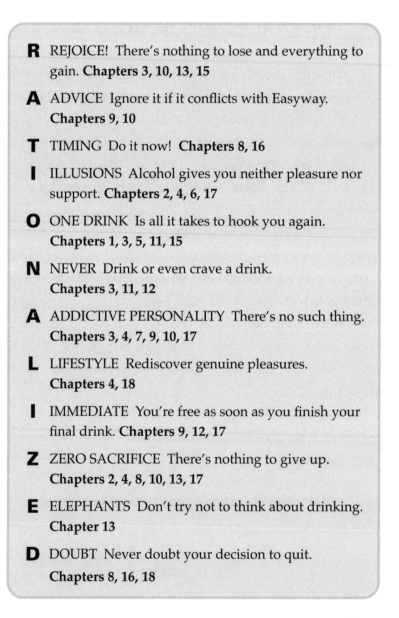

**R** REJOICE! There's nothing to lose and everything to gain. **Chapters 3, 10, 13, 15**

**A** ADVICE  Ignore it if it conflicts with Easyway. **Chapters 9, 10**

**T** TIMING  Do it now!  **Chapters 8, 16**

**I** ILLUSIONS  Alcohol gives you neither pleasure nor support. **Chapters 2, 4, 6, 17**

**O** ONE DRINK  Is all it takes to hook you again. **Chapters 1, 3, 5, 11, 15**

**N** NEVER  Drink or even crave a drink. **Chapters 3, 11, 12**

**A** ADDICTIVE PERSONALITY  There's no such thing. **Chapters 3, 4, 7, 9, 10, 17**

**L** LIFESTYLE  Rediscover genuine pleasures. **Chapters 4, 18**

**I** IMMEDIATE  You're free as soon as you finish your final drink. **Chapters 9, 12, 17**

**Z** ZERO SACRIFICE  There's nothing to give up. **Chapters 2, 4, 8, 10, 13, 17**

**E** ELEPHANTS  Don't try not to think about drinking. **Chapter 13**

**D** DOUBT  Never doubt your decision to quit. **Chapters 8, 16, 18**

If you understand the nature of the trap and you're eager and have no doubts about walking free, there's no reason to delay. If you're hesitating, please go through the RATIONALIZED list again or contact your nearest Allen Carr's Easyway To Stop Drinking Center if you have any questions.

## SUMMARY

- The ideal time to stop is now. There is no reason to wait.
- Go through the checklist and if you're missing anything, go back and reread the relevant chapters.

# Chapter 17

# YOUR FINAL DRINK

## IN THIS CHAPTER
• *LAST-MINUTE NERVES*
• *THE RITUAL*
• *NEVER MIND THE OUTCOME*

*The vow never to drink again marks the breaking point in the cycle of addiction. It's important that you observe the ritual— as soon as you complete it, you're free.*

And so the time has come. You're about to escape from one of the most subtle and insidious traps ever devised. All along I've promised you it would be easy, but that shouldn't diminish your sense of achievement in any way. To go through the method as instructed, and understand the nature of the trap, requires considerable discipline and perseverance. It also takes courage to open your mind. Be proud of your achievement. You've reached a position that millions of drinkers wish they could achieve.

If you feel nervous, don't worry about it. That's completely normal at this stage and is no threat to your chances of success. When you make a parachute jump, the last-minute nerves quickly turn to exhilaration as your parachute opens and you realize that everything you've learned and prepared for is working exactly how they told you it would. I wish I could put into words the utter joy of the person who has finally accepted that they don't need to drink any more.

The elation is unbelievable. It's like a huge, dark shadow being removed from your mind. You no longer need to despise yourself, or have to worry about what it's been doing to your health, or all the money that you waste.

You no longer have to worry about where the next drink is coming from. You'll no longer feel weak, miserable, sordid, incomplete, or guilty.

You're in that position now, standing by the plane door, ready to jump. You have all the knowledge and understanding you need to make this the best experience of your life. Soon you will be flying free. You have nothing to fear. The only thing that is facing sudden death is your drinking problem. You are not losing a friend; you have no reason to grieve. On the contrary, you should rejoice in the destruction of your mortal enemy.

Remind yourself that you're not "giving up" anything. You had no need to drink before you started; you have no need to drink now. Lifelong nondrinkers and ex-drinkers are quite happy without drinking. What pleasure does it give? What support does it provide? If you've followed and understood everything up to this point, you'll have come to the obvious conclusion:

### *THERE IS NO REASON TO DRINK*

**IN HER OWN WORDS: SARAH**

I'm overjoyed. I recently quit drinking with Easyway and I know I'll never touch another drink. It's opened my eyes to so many things: I now realize I didn't even enjoy drinking, but my addiction made me neglect other important areas of my life: my children, my health, my home. I feel all the benefits that Allen mentioned: I feel healthy, full of energy, and I've learned to respect myself again. No more self-loathing. I'm in control and I've been told by my husband that the change in my mood is amazing. Thank you, Allen. I can't wait to get on with my life now.

Very soon I'll ask you to take your final drink and make a solemn vow never to drink again. Before you do, it's essential you're completely reconciled with the notion of never drinking again. You must be absolutely clear that drinking gives you no pleasure or support whatsoever and you're not making any sort of sacrifice.

If you find the thought of never having another drink difficult to accept, try taking on board the only alternative: spending the rest of your life drinking, never being allowed to stop.

It's a simple choice. If you still feel as if you're being made to choose the lesser of two evils, ask yourself this: Does it concern you that you might never suffer from flu again, or you might never suffer from AIDS, or that you might never inject yourself with heroin?

No? Then why should it bother you that you will never again suffer at the hands of one of the world's biggest killers? Alcohol addiction is a disease. It started when you began to consume the addictive poison. It ends when you finish your final drink.

It's ridiculously easy to stop drinking provided you understand there's nothing to give up and you follow all the instructions. You're stopping because you detest being a slave to alcohol. So instead of thinking, "I must never drink again," start thinking, "This is great! I don't ever need to waste my time and money on making myself miserable again. I'M FREE!"

## THE RITUAL

This is a momentous occasion and one of the most important decisions you'll ever make. You're freeing yourself from slavery and achieving something great, something all drinkers would love to achieve and something that everybody, drinkers and nondrinkers alike, will admire and respect you for. What's more, you'll go right up in the estimations of one person in particular: yourself.

You should now be feeling excited about finally ending the misery that drinking has caused you. You may be wondering whether you actually want to bother with the ritual of the final drink. Some people have what they hope will be their final drink before opening this book and by the time they reach this stage they're adamant that they have no desire ever to drink again. If this applies to you, it's good news because it means you have fully removed the desire to drink. If you've already stopped, do not take another drink now; you have already had your final drink, but do make the vow never to drink again.

The thing that makes it difficult to quit is not the physical aggravation of withdrawal; it's the doubt, the uncertainty, the waiting to become a nondrinker. With this method, you become a nondrinker the moment you finish your final drink and you make your vow never to drink again. It's important to know when that moment is, to be able to make that vow with a feeling of venom, to visualize your triumph over the Little Monster and be able to say, "Yes! I'm a nondrinker now. I'm FREE!"

Your mindset at this moment should be one of certainty. It's not enough to hope that you will never drink again; you need to know. So let's just go over the things that may cause you to doubt your decision:

1. The belief that you're making a genuine sacrifice.

Get it clearly into your mind:

### THERE IS ABSOLUTELY NOTHING TO GIVE UP

Drinking gives no genuine pleasure or support whatsoever. The fact that it appears to is just an illusion.

2. The belief that it's possible to have the occasional drink without getting hooked.

Remember:

### THERE IS ONLY ONE ESSENTIAL TO BEING A NONDRINKER AND THAT IS NOT TO DRINK—EVER

## *IN ORDER TO BE A HAPPY NONDRINKER FOR LIFE, IT'S ESSENTIAL NEVER TO DESIRE TO DRINK*

If you have a desire to have just one drink, you'll have a desire to have another and another. Get it clearly into your mind: It has to be all or nothing.

There are two other factors that can make you doubt your decision:

3.  The belief that you're a confirmed drinker, or have an addictive personality.

Anyone can fall for the alcohol trap—and most people do. Even if you did have an addictive personality, that would simply mean that you easily get addicted; it would not mean that you would find it difficult to stop.

4.  The influence of other drinkers.

They're the ones who are losing out, not you. If you have read and understood this book, you have infinitely more expertise on the subject than they have. Don't envy them, pity them. They're still in the trap; you are escaping.

## THE FINAL DRINK

You are about to make the decision to have your final drink and never to consume alcohol again.

If you made that decision before you picked up this book, you need to reconfirm the decision in your mind now. This is the moment when you walk free. Think about the misery and suffering that alcohol has caused you. Visualize the Little Monster and how it has dominated your life. Imagine it laughing at you. This is the time for your revenge. Make your vow. No more slavery! No more misery! You're cutting off its lifeline and destroying that evil tyrant once and for all.

### *I WOULD LIKE YOU NOW TO CONSUME YOUR FINAL DRINK. REJOICE! YOU'RE FREE!*

Revel in your victory. This is one of the greatest achievements of your life. It's important that this moment sticks in your mind. Be aware that at the moment you're fired up with powerful reasons to stop, but as the days, weeks, and years slip by, your memory of how you were feeling about drinking today may dim. Implant those thoughts in your mind now while they're vivid, so that even if your memory of the details should diminish, your resolution never to drink again does not.

### FOREWARNED IS FOREARMED

If you're prepared for a challenge, it doesn't faze you as it would if it took you completely by surprise. You can easily guard against any moments of doubt in the future by having the foresight to plan ahead.

In a few months you'll find it difficult to believe that you once found it necessary to drink alcohol, let alone how it controlled your life. You may also lose your fear of getting hooked again. Be aware now, in advance, that this can be a danger; you might have moments when you're on a high, surrounded by drinkers, or you might suffer a trauma and your guard will be down. Anticipate these situations now and make it part of your vow that, if and when they come, you will be prepared, so that there is no way that you'll be fooled into starting to drink again. Keep it clearly in your mind that alcohol neither made the good times better nor relieved stress during the bad times. It did the complete opposite.

Now you can move on. Don't wait for anything. Embrace this moment with a feeling of excitement and elation. The nightmare is over.

### *FREEDOM STARTS HERE!*

Congratulations! You're ready to start enjoying life as a nondrinker!

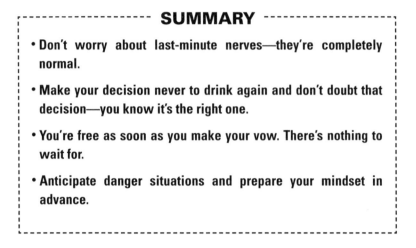

**SUMMARY**

• Don't worry about last-minute nerves—they're completely normal.

• Make your decision never to drink again and don't doubt that decision—you know it's the right one.

• You're free as soon as you make your vow. There's nothing to wait for.

• Anticipate danger situations and prepare your mindset in advance.

# Chapter 18

# ENJOYING LIFE FREE FROM ALCOHOL

## IN THIS CHAPTER
*•THE FIRST FEW DAYS  •ALL YOU HAVE GAINED*
*•COPING WITH BAD DAYS*
*•STAYING FREE FOREVER*

*You've done it! You're now a nondrinker and will remain one permanently provided you never doubt your decision.*

You become a nondrinker the moment you finish your final drink. You can immediately get on with the rest of your life and enjoying the many pleasures it has to offer. For a few days after your final drink, you may detect the cries of the Little Monster as it goes through its death throes. This is nothing to worry about, so don't try to block it from your mind. Recognize the cries and rejoice in what they signify—the death of the monster that has held you enslaved for all this time.

As a drinker you felt compelled to feed the Little Monster. Now you're free, you don't have to do anything. That's the method for killing the Little Monster:

### *DO NOTHING!*

I told you it was easy.

With the willpower method, no one tells you that the death throes are a sign that you've won. Instead they're taken as evidence of what you always feared: that quitting will be hard. Rather than rejoicing at the death of the Little Monster, people who try to quit with willpower respond in various negative ways: feeling irritable, restless, angry, insecure, disorientated, or lethargic. They allow these feelings to make them think they might be better off drinking again. They forget that they already suffered from these feelings throughout their drinking lives; they're the same feelings that they always interpreted as "I want a drink."

Living with the death throes is no harder than living with a mild cold and they only last for a few days. They only become a problem if you start to worry about them or interpret them as a need or desire to drink. If you feel them, picture a Little Monster searching around the desert for a drink and you having control of the water supply. All you have to do is keep the tap closed. It's as easy as that.

Prepare your mindset in advance so that you're ready with the right response. Instead of thinking, "I want a drink but I'm not allowed one," think, "This is the Little Monster demanding its fix. This is what drinkers suffer throughout their drinking lives. Nondrinkers don't suffer this feeling. Isn't it great! I'm a nondrinker and so I'll soon be free of it forever." Remind yourself that there is no physical pain and that the only discomfort you might be feeling is not because you've stopped drinking but because you started in the first place. Also be clear that having another drink, far from relieving that discomfort, would insure that you suffered it for the rest of your life.

Prepare your mind to respond in this way and any withdrawal pangs will become moments of pleasure. Revel in the Little Monster's death throes. Feel no guilt about rejoicing in its death; after all, it's been killing you, making you miserable, and keeping you a slave for long enough.

## YOUR NEW LIFE STARTS HERE

People trying to quit with the willpower method are forever moping for something they hope they'll never do, forever waiting for nothing to happen. But when you have no desire to drink, you don't have to wait or mope for anything. You don't have to stand by and grit your teeth while the Little Monster dies; you can get straight on with enjoying life as a nondrinker.

One of the fantastic benefits of becoming a nondrinker is that you rediscover the joy of life's genuine pleasures. When you're addicted to alcohol you lose the ability fully to enjoy the things that nondrinkers enjoy most: reading books, getting out and about, watching entertainment, social occasions, exercise, sex… now that you're a nondrinker, you have all these pleasures to get excited about.

You will find that situations you have come to regard as unstimulating or even irritating become enjoyable again: things like spending time with your loved ones, going for walks, seeing friends. Work too will become more enjoyable, as you find you're better able to concentrate, to think creatively, and to handle stress.

At the same time, you become more discerning about the things you don't like. When I stopped drinking I realized I had wasted a lot of time going to boring functions that gave me no pleasure at all. I would go and I would drink, thinking that would help me relax and enjoy the occasion. But when I stopped I was able to see that it wasn't a failure on my part that those occasions seemed boring—they were boring. So I stopped going to them, or if I had to go, I would make my excuses and leave at the first opportunity. When you cut alcohol out of your life, you regain the ability to see things as they really are and make better decisions about how you run your life.

## WHEN THE CLOUDS GATHER

Be prepared for bad days. Everybody, drinker and nondrinker alike, has bad days when everything that can go wrong seems to. It has nothing to do with the fact that you've stopped drinking. The truth is, when you stop drinking you find the bad days don't come around so frequently, and when they do, you feel stronger to cope with them.

You might well find that when you have bad days the thought of drinking enters your mind. That's not unusual and it's nothing to worry about. You don't have to push the thought out of your mind, you just have to recognize it for what it is: a remnant from the days when you responded to every setback by drinking. It doesn't mean you're still vulnerable to the trap. It just means you're still adjusting to your newfound freedom. Rather than thinking, "I mustn't drink", or, "I thought I'd overcome this addiction", think,

"Great! I don't have to drink any more. I'm free!"

The thought will pass very quickly and your brain will soon adjust. It's essential that you never doubt or question your decision to stop. Never make the mistake that people on the willpower method make, of craving another drink. If you do you will put yourself in the same impossible position as them: miserable if you don't and even more miserable if you do.

My final instruction is one that you have already decided for yourself:

### *NEVER DRINK ALCOHOL AGAIN!*

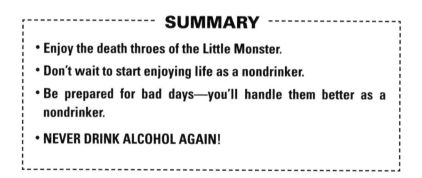

---- **SUMMARY** ----

- Enjoy the death throes of the Little Monster.
- Don't wait to start enjoying life as a nondrinker.
- Be prepared for bad days—you'll handle them better as a nondrinker.
- NEVER DRINK ALCOHOL AGAIN!

# Chapter 19

# USEFUL REMINDERS

*From time to time you may find it useful to remind yourself of some of the issues that we've discussed. Here I've summarized the key points, together with a reminder of the instructions. Follow these and you will remain a happy nondrinker for the rest of your life.*

- Don't wait for anything. You're already a nondrinker from the moment you finish your final drink. You've cut off the supply to the Little Monster and unlocked the door of your prison.

- Accept that there will always be good days and bad days. Because you will be stronger both physically and mentally, within no time at all you'll enjoy the good times more and handle the bad times better.

- Be aware that a very important change is happening in your life. Like all major changes, including those for the better, it can take a little time for your mind and body to adjust. Don't worry if you feel different or disorientated for a few days. Just accept it.

- Remember you've stopped drinking, you haven't stopped living. You can now start enjoying life to the full.

- There is no need to avoid other drinkers. Go out and enjoy social occasions and show yourself you can handle them right from the start.

- Don't envy drinkers. When you're with them, remind yourself you're not being deprived; they are.

- Never doubt or question your decision to stop—you know it's the right one. Never crave another drink. If you do, you will put yourself in an impossible position: You will be miserable if you don't and even more miserable if you do.

- Make sure right from the start that if the thought of "just one drink" enters your mind, you think, "YIPPEE! I'm a nondrinker." The thought will pass very quickly from your brain and it will quickly learn not to think it again.

- Don't try not to think about drinking. It's impossible to make your brain not think about something. By trying to, you will make yourself frustrated and miserable. It's easy to think about drinking without feeling miserable: Instead of thinking, "I mustn't drink," or, "When will the craving go?" think, "Great! I'm a nondrinker. Yippee! I'm free!"

## THE INSTRUCTIONS

1.  Follow all the instructions in order.

2.  Keep an open mind.

3.  Start with a feeling of elation.

4.  Never doubt your decision to quit. You know it's the right one.

5.  Ignore all advice and influences that conflict with Easyway.

6.  Don't wait to quit. Do it now!

7.  Never drink alcohol again!

# Chapter 20

# THE HYPNOTHERAPY

This book comes with an audio hypnotherapy session.

You can listen to the audio by visiting this link
**https://delivr.com/2tj9u** or by scanning the QR code below.

The hypnotherapy is specifically for use with this book.
It will not be effective unless you have already read the book
and drunk your final drink.

**Warning: Do not listen to this recording while driving or
operating heavy machinery or if you suffer from epilepsy.
If in doubt consult your doctor.**

Although Allen Carr's Easyway centers have always used an element of hypnotherapy as part of the process, it's important to stress that it's not the hypnotherapy itself that enables drinkers, smokers, or other addicts to quit. The key to the method is removing the illusions brought about by brainwashing. In this case, it means removing the illusion that alcohol gives you any benefit or pleasure.

Hypnotherapy can be a helpful tool in this process, but it's misleading to say that hypnotherapy can stop you from drinking, just as it's misleading to say a book can stop you. It's too simplistic. The key lies in the content of the book—and in the content of the hypnotherapy.

A farmer trying to raise crops in an arid part of the world will be thankful for the pipeline that brings water to irrigate his land, but it isn't the pipeline that makes his crops grow; it's the water within it. If the pipeline was carrying oil it would be useless to the farmer. Hypnotherapy is like a pipeline: It's only of use if its content is right.

You have received the content by reading this book and now the hypnotherapy is going to help you absorb it. If you haven't yet read the book, please do so before you listen to the hypnotherapy. It's important that you use the hypnotherapy and the book together. The hypnotherapy is completely different from the live experience at Allen Carr's Easyway centers. It's designed to work as an additional tool to help you absorb the contents of the book, and it will only be effective if you have read the book beforehand.

You may be thinking that you've absorbed all the key messages by reading the book and that you have no need to listen to the hypnotherapy. Perhaps that's true, but I would still advise you to listen to the hypnotherapy because it will help you to take in all the information you've read in a relaxing and effective way, without any distractions or interruptions.

Easyway centers are specially designed to provide an environment that is geared toward comfort and relaxation. The rooms are furnished with comfortable chairs, lighting is soft, and the temperature is maintained at a pleasant level.

Visitors are much more likely to absorb all the information we give them if they're relaxed and not distracted by anything. The mind is much more receptive when it's in this relaxed state. All you have to do is sit back and take it all in. So listen to the hypnotherapy in a similar environment.

However, it's not uncommon to be apprehensive about hypnotherapy. People talk about "going under," being "put to sleep," or "losing control." I can reassure you:

### NOTHING WEIRD IS GOING TO HAPPEN

You will remain in control throughout the hypnotherapy and there will be no ill effects whatsoever. Some people do drift off to sleep during hypnosis, and that is fine because their unconscious mind will still hear and take in the message. But if an emergency were to arise, rest assured that you would respond as normal, even if you have drifted off to sleep. You have absolutely nothing to be concerned about.

The aim, however, is not to drift off to sleep but just to relax. You may experience a floating feeling or a warm, embracing feeling of deep relaxation, and your thoughts may wander blissfully as if in a daydream. If so, lucky you. This is a lovely state to be in and highly conducive to absorbing new ideas.

If you don't feel yourself drifting off at all, don't worry: It doesn't mean it's not working. Most people report that nothing much seems to happen, but the hypnotherapy still works for them. All that is required of you is to be nicely relaxed and ready to absorb all the messages that will insure that you solve your drinking problem and start enjoying a new life free from the slavery of alcohol addiction.

*THE HYPNOTHERAPY WILL NOT BE EFFECTIVE UNLESS YOU HAVE ALREADY READ THE BOOK. IF YOU HAVE NOT ALREADY DONE SO, PLEASE DO SO BEFORE YOU LISTEN TO THE HYPNOTHERAPY*

## LIST OF ALLEN CARR'S EASYWAY CENTERS

The following list indicates the countries where Allen Carr's Easyway To Stop Smoking Centers are currently operational.

Check www.allencarr.com for latest additions to this list.

The success rate at the centers, based on the three-month money-back guarantee, is over 90 percent.

Selected centers also offer sessions that deal with alcohol, other drugs and weight issues. Please check with your nearest center, listed below, for details.

Allen Carr's Easyway guarantee that you will find it easy to stop at the centers or your money back.

## JOIN US!

Allen Carr's Easyway Centers have spread throughout the world with incredible speed and success. Our global franchise network now covers more than 150 cities in over 45 countries. This amazing growth has been achieved entirely organically. Former addicts, just like you, were so impressed by the ease with which they stopped that they felt inspired to contact us to see how they could bring the method to their region.

If you feel the same, contact us for details on how to become an Allen Carr's Easyway To Stop Smoking or an Allen Carr's Easyway To Stop Drinking franchisee.

Email us at: **join-us@allencarr.com** including your full name, postal address, and region of interest.

## SUPPORT US!

No, don't send us money!

You have achieved something really marvelous. Every time we hear of someone escaping from the sinking ship, we get a feeling of enormous satisfaction.

It would give us great pleasure to hear that you have freed yourself from the slavery of addiction so please visit the following web page where you can tell us of your success, inspire others to follow in your footsteps, and hear about ways you can help to spread the word.

**www.allencarr.com/fanzone**

You can "like" our facebook page here
**www.facebook.com/AllenCarr**

Together, we can help further Allen Carr's mission: to cure the world of addiction.

# ALLEN CARR'S EASYWAY CENTERS

### LONDON CLINIC AND WORLDWIDE HEAD OFFICE

Park House, 14 Pepys Road, Raynes Park, London SW20 8NH

Tel: +44 (0)20 8944 7761

Fax: +44 (0)20 8944 8619

Email: mail@allencarr.com

Website: www.allencarr.com

Therapists: John Dicey, Colleen Dwyer, Crispin Hay, Emma Hudson, Rob Fielding, Sam Kelser, Rob Groves, Debbie Brewer-West, Mark Keen, Duncan Bhaskaran-Brown, Mark Newman, Gerry Williams (Alcohol) Monique Douglas (Weight)

### WORLDWIDE PRESS OFFICE

Tel: +44 (0)7970 88 44 52

Contact: John Dicey

Tel: +44 (0)7970 88 44 52

Email: media@allencarr.com

# NORTH AMERICAN CENTERS

### U.S.A.

Sessions held throughout the USA

Tel: +1 855 440 3777

Email: support@usa.allencarr.com

Website: www.allencarr.com

### New York

Tel: +1 855 440 3777

Therapists: Natalie Clays and Team

Email: support@usa.allencarr.com

Website: www.allencarr.com

### Los Angeles

Tel: +1 855 440 3777

Therapists: Natalie Clays and Team

Email: support@usa.allencarr.com

Website: www.allencarr.com

### Milwaukee (and South Wisconsin)

Tel: +1 262 770 1260

Therapist: Wayne Spaulding

Email: wayne@easywaywisconsin.com

Website: www.allencarr.com

### CANADA

Tel: +1 855 440 3777

Therapist: Natalie Clays

Email: natalie@ca.allencarr.com

Website: www.allencarr.com

# U.K. CENTERS

UK Clinic Information and Central Booking Line

Tel: 0800 389 2115 (UK only)

## Birmingham

Tel & Fax: 0800 389 2115
Therapists: John Dicey, Colleen Dwyer, Crispin Hay, Emma Hudson, Rob Fielding, Sam Kelser, Rob Groves, Debbie Brewer-West, Mark Keen, Duncan Bhaskaran-Brown, Mark Newman
Email: mail@allencarr.com
Website: www.allencarr.com

## Bournemouth

Tel: 0800 389 2115
Therapists: John Dicey, Colleen Dwyer, Crispin Hay, Emma Hudson, Rob Fielding, Sam Kelser, Rob Groves, Debbie Brewer-West, Mark Keen, Duncan Bhaskaran-Brown, Mark Newman
Email: mail@allencarr.com
Website: www.allencarr.com

## Brentwood

Tel: 0800 389 2115
Therapists: John Dicey, Colleen Dwyer, Crispin Hay, Emma Hudson, Rob Fielding, Sam Kelser, Rob Groves, Debbie Brewer-West, Mark Keen, Duncan Bhaskaran-Brown, Mark Newman
Email: mail@allencarr.com
Website: www.allencarr.com

## Brighton

Tel: 0800 389 2115
Therapists: John Dicey, Colleen Dwyer, Crispin Hay, Emma Hudson, Rob Fielding, Sam Kelser, Rob Groves, Debbie Brewer-West, Mark Keen, Duncan Bhaskaran-Brown, Mark Newman
Email: mail@allencarr.com
Website: www.allencarr.com

## Bristol

Tel: 0800 389 2115
Therapists: John Dicey, Colleen Dwyer, Crispin Hay, Emma Hudson, Rob Fielding, Sam Kelser, Rob Groves, Debbie Brewer-West, Mark Keen, Duncan Bhaskaran-Brown, Mark Newman
Email: mail@allencarr.com
Website: www.allencarr.com

## Cambridge

Tel: 0800 389 2115
Therapists: John Dicey, Colleen Dwyer, Crispin Hay, Emma Hudson, Rob Fielding, Sam Kelser, Rob Groves, Debbie Brewer-West, Mark Keen, Duncan Bhaskaran-Brown, Mark Newman
Email: mail@allencarr.com
Website: www.allencarr.com

## Coventry

Tel: 0800 321 3007
Therapist: Rob Fielding
Email: info@easywaymidlands.co.uk
Website: www.allencarr.com

## Cumbria

Tel: 0800 389 2115
Therapists: John Dicey, Colleen
Dwyer, Crispin Hay, Emma
Hudson, Rob Fielding, Sam Kelser,
Rob Groves, Debbie Brewer-West,
Mark Keen, Duncan Bhaskaran-
Brown, Mark Newman
Email: mail@allencarr.com
Website: www.allencarr.com

## Derby

Tel: 0800 389 2115
Therapists: John Dicey, Colleen
Dwyer, Crispin Hay, Emma
Hudson, Rob Fielding, Sam Kelser,
Rob Groves, Debbie Brewer-West,
Mark Keen, Duncan Bhaskaran-
Brown, Mark Newman
Email: mail@allencarr.com
Website: www.allencarr.com

## Guernsey

Tel: 0800 077 6187
Therapist: Mark Keen
Email:
mark@easywaymanchester.co.uk
Website: www.allencarr.com

## Isle of Man

Tel: 0800 077 6187
Therapist: Mark Keen
Email:
mark@easywaymanchester.co.uk
Website: www.allencarr.com

## Jersey

Tel: 0800 077 6187
Therapist: Mark Keen
Email:
mark@easywaymanchester.co.uk
Website: www.allencarr.com

## Kent

Tel: 0800 389 2115
Therapists: John Dicey, Colleen
Dwyer, Crispin Hay, Emma
Hudson, Rob Fielding, Sam Kelser,
Rob Groves, Debbie Brewer-West,
Mark Keen, Duncan Bhaskaran-
Brown, Mark Newman
Email: mail@allencarr.com
Website: www.allencarr.com

## Lancashire

Tel: 0800 389 2115
Therapists: John Dicey, Colleen
Dwyer, Crispin Hay, Emma
Hudson, Rob Fielding, Sam Kelser,
Rob Groves, Debbie Brewer-West,
Mark Keen, Duncan Bhaskaran-
Brown, Mark Newman
Email: mail@allencarr.com
Website: www.allencarr.com

## Leeds

Tel: 0800 077 6187
Therapist: Mark Keen
Email:
mark@easywaymanchester.co.uk
Website: www.allencarr.com

## Leicester

Tel: 0800 321 3007
Therapist: Rob Fielding
Email:
info@easywaymidlands.co.uk
Website: www.allencarr.com

## Lincoln

Tel: 0800 321 3007
Therapist: Rob Fielding
Email:
info@easywaymidlands.co.uk
Website: www.allencarr.com

## Liverpool

Tel: 0800 389 2115
Therapists: John Dicey, Colleen
Dwyer, Crispin Hay, Emma
Hudson, Rob Fielding, Sam Kelser,
Rob Groves, Debbie Brewer-West,
Mark Keen, Duncan Bhaskaran-
Brown, Mark Newman
Email: mail@allencarr.com
Website: www.allencarr.com

## Manchester

Tel: 0800 077 6187
Therapist: Mark Keen
Email:
mark@easywaymanchester.co.uk
Website: www.allencarr.com

## Milton Keynes

Tel: 0800 389 2115
Therapists: John Dicey, Colleen
Dwyer, Crispin Hay, Emma
Hudson, Rob Fielding, Sam Kelser,
Rob Groves, Debbie Brewer-West,
Mark Keen, Duncan Bhaskaran-
Brown, Mark Newman
Email: mail@allencarr.com
Website: www.allencarr.com

## Newcastle/North East

Tel: 0800 389 2115
Therapists: John Dicey, Colleen
Dwyer, Crispin Hay, Emma
Hudson, Rob Fielding, Sam Kelser,
Rob Groves, Debbie Brewer-West,
Mark Keen, Duncan Bhaskaran-
Brown, Mark Newman
Email:
mail@allencarr.com
Website: www.allencarr.com

## Nottingham

Tel: 0800 389 2115
Therapists:John Dicey, Colleen
Dwyer, Crispin Hay, Emma
Hudson, Rob Fielding, Sam Kelser,
Rob Groves, Debbie Brewer-West,
Mark Keen, Duncan Bhaskaran-
Brown, Mark Newman
Email: mail@allencarr.com
Website: www.allencarr.com

## Oxford

Tel: 0800 389 2115
Therapists: John Dicey, Colleen
Dwyer, Crispin Hay, Emma
Hudson, Rob Fielding, Sam Kelser,
Rob Groves, Debbie Brewer-West,
Mark Keen, Duncan Bhaskaran-
Brown, Mark Newman
Email: mail@allencarr.com
Website: www.allencarr.com

## Reading

Tel: 0800 389 2115
Therapists: John Dicey, Colleen
Dwyer, Crispin Hay, Emma
Hudson, Rob Fielding, Sam Kelser,
Rob Groves, Debbie Brewer-West,
Mark Keen, Duncan Bhaskaran-
Brown, Mark Newman
Email: mail@allencarr.com
Website: www.allencarr.com

## SCOTLAND
## Glasgow and Edinburgh

Tel: +44 (0)131 449 7858
Therapists: Paul Melvin and Jim
McCreadie
Email: info@easywayscotland.co.uk
Website: www.allencarr.com

## Southampton

Tel: 0800 389 2115
Therapists: John Dicey, Colleen
Dwyer, Crispin Hay, Emma
Hudson, Rob Fielding, Sam Kelser,
Rob Groves, Debbie Brewer-West,
Mark Keen, Duncan Bhaskaran-
Brown, Mark Newman
Email: mail@allencarr.com
Website: www.allencarr.com

## Southport

Tel: 0800 389 2115
Therapists: John Dicey, Colleen
Dwyer, Crispin Hay, Emma
Hudson, Rob Fielding, Sam Kelser,
Rob Groves, Debbie Brewer-West,
Mark Keen, Duncan Bhaskaran-
Brown, Mark Newman
Email: mail@allencarr.com
Website: www.allencarr.com

## Staines/Heathrow

Tel: 0800 389 2115
Therapists: John Dicey, Colleen
Dwyer, Crispin Hay, Emma
Hudson, Rob Fielding, Sam Kelser,
Rob Groves, Debbie Brewer-West,
Mark Keen, Duncan Bhaskaran-
Brown, Mark Newman
Email: mail@allencarr.com
Website: www.allencarr.com

## Stevenage

Tel: 0800 389 2115
Therapists: John Dicey, Colleen
Dwyer, Crispin Hay, Emma
Hudson, Rob Fielding, Sam Kelser,
Rob Groves, Debbie Brewer-West,
Mark Keen, Duncan Bhaskaran-
Brown, Mark Newman
Email: mail@allencarr.com
Website: www.allencarr.com

## Stoke

Tel: 0800 389 2115
Therapists: John Dicey, Colleen
Dwyer, Crispin Hay, Emma
Hudson, Rob Fielding, Sam Kelser,
Rob Groves, Debbie Brewer-West,
Mark Keen, Duncan Bhaskaran-
Brown, Mark Newman
Email: mail@allencarr.com
Website: www.allencarr.com

## Surrey

Park House, 14 Pepys Road, Raynes
Park, London SW20 8NH
Tel: +44 (0)20 8944 7761
Fax: +44 (0)20 8944 8619
Therapists: John Dicey, Colleen
Dwyer, Crispin Hay, Emma
Hudson, Rob Fielding, Sam Kelser,
Rob Groves, Debbie Brewer-West,

Mark Keen, Duncan Bhaskaran-Brown, Mark Newman
Gerry Williams (Alcohol), Monique Douglas (Weight)
Email: mail@allencarr.com
Website: www.allencarr.com

## Watford
Tel: 0800 389 2115
Therapists: John Dicey, Colleen Dwyer, Crispin Hay, Emma Hudson, Rob Fielding, Sam Kelser, Rob Groves, Debbie Brewer-West, Mark Keen, Duncan Bhaskaran-Brown, Mark Newman
Email: mail@allencarr.com
Website: www.allencarr.com

## Worcester
Tel: 0800 321 3007
Therapist: Rob Fielding
Email: info@easywaymidlands.co.uk
Website: www.allencarr.com

# WORLDWIDE CENTERS

## AUSTRALIA
### ACT, NSW, NT, QLD, VIC
Tel: 1300 848 028
Therapist: Natalie Clays and Team
Email: natalie@allencarr.com.au
Website: www.allencarr.com

### South Australia
Tel: 1300 848 028
Therapist: Jaime Reed
Email: sa@allencarr.com.au
Website: www.allencarr.com

### Western Australia
Tel: 1300 848 028
Therapist: Natalie Clays and Team
Email: natalie@allencarr.com.au
Website: www.allencarr.com

## AUSTRIA
Sessions held throughout Austria
Freephone: 0800RAUCHEN
(0800 7282436)
Tel: +43 (0)3512 44755
Therapists: Erich Kellermann and Team
Email: info@allen-carr.at
Website: www.allencarr.com

## BELGIUM
### Brussels
Tel: +32 (0)2 808 19 65
Therapist: Paula Rooduijn
Email: info@allencarr.be
Website: www.allencarr.com

## BRAZIL
Therapist : Lilian Brunstein
Email: contato@easywayonline.com.br
Website: www.allencarr.com

## BULGARIA
Tel: 0800 14104/+359 899 88 99 07
Therapist: Rumyana Kostadinova
Email: rk@nepushaveche.com
Website: www.allencarr.com

## CHILE
Tel: +56 2 4744587
Therapist: Claudia Sarmiento
Email: contacto@allencarr.cl
Website: www.allencarr.com

## CYPRUS

Tel: +357 25770611
Therapist: Andreas Damianou
Email: info@allencarr.com.cy
Website: www.allencarr.com

## DENMARK

Sessions held throughout Denmark
Tel: +45 70267711
Therapist: Mette Fønss
Email: mette@easyway.dk
Website: www.allencarr.com

## ESTONIA

Tel: +372 733 0044
Therapist: Henry Jakobson
Email: info@allencarr.ee
Website: www.allencarr.com

## FINLAND

Tel: +358-(0)45 3544099
Therapist: Janne Ström
Email: info@allencarr.fi
Website: www.allencarr.com

## FRANCE

Sessions held throughout France
Freephone: 0800 386387
Tel: +33 (4) 91 33 54 55
Therapists: Erick Serre and Team
Email: info@allencarr.fr
Website: www.allencarr.com

## GERMANY

Sessions held throughout Germany
Freephone: 08000RAUCHEN
(0800 07282436)
Tel: +49 (0) 8031 90190-0
Therapists: Erich Kellermann
and Team
Email: info@allen-carr.de
Website: www.allencarr.com

## GREECE

Sessions held throughout Greece
Tel: +30 210 5224087
Therapist: Panos Tzouras
Email: panos@allencarr.gr
Website: www.allencarr.com

## GUATEMALA

Tel: +502 2362 0000
Therapist: Michelle Binford
Email:
info@dejadefumarfacil.com
Website: www.allencarr.com

## HONG KONG

Email: info@easywayhongkong.com
Website: www.allencarr.com

## HUNGARY

Seminars in Budapest and
12 other cities across Hungary
Tel: 06 80 624 426 (freephone) or
+36 20 580 9244
Therapist: Gábor Szász
Email: szasz.gabor@allencarr.hu
Website: www.allencarr.com

## INDIA
### Bangalore and Chennai

Tel: +91 (0)80 4154 0624
Therapist: Suresh Shottam
Email: info@
easywaytostopsmoking.co.in
Website: www.allencarr.com

## IRAN

Please check website for details
Tehran and Mshhad
Website: www.allencarr.com

## ISRAEL

Sessions held throughout Israel
Tel: +972 (0)3 6212525
Therapists: Orit Rozen and Team
Email: info@allencarr.co.il
Website: www.allencarr.com

## ITALY

Sessions held throughout Italy
Tel/Fax: +39 (0)2 7060 2438
Therapists: Francesca Cesati and Team
Email: info@easywayitalia.com
Website: www.allencarr.com

## JAPAN

Sessions held throughout Japan
www.allencarr.com

## LEBANON

Tel: +961 1 791 5565
Therapist: Sadek El-Assaad
Email: info@AllenCarrEasyWay.me
Website: www.allencarr.com

## MAURITIUS

Tel: +230 5727 5103
Therapist: Heidi Hoareau
Email: info@allencarr.mu
Website: www.allencarr.com

## MEXICO

Sessions held throughout Mexico
Tel: +52 55 2623 0631
Therapists: Jorge Davo and Team
Email: info@allencarr-mexico.com
Website: www.allencarr.com

## NETHERLANDS

Sessions held throughout the
Netherlands
Allen Carr's Easyway
'stoppen met roken'
Tel: +31 53 478 43 62/
+31 900 786 77 37
Email: info@allencarr.nl
Website: www.allencarr.com

## NEW ZEALAND
### North Island – Auckland

Tel: +64 (0) 800 848 028
Therapist: Natalie Clays and Team
Email: natalie@allencarr.co.nz
Website: www.allencarr.com

### South Island – Wellington and Christchurch

Tel: +64 (0) 800 848 028
Therapist: Natalie Clays and Team
Email: natalie@allencarr.co.nz

## NORWAY

Therapist: Laila Thorsen
Please check website for details
Website: www.allencarr.com

## PERU
### Lima

Tel: +511 637 7310
Therapist: Luis Loranca
Email: lloranca@
dejardefumaraltoque.com
Website: www.allencarr.com

## POLAND

Sessions held throughout Poland
Tel: +48 (0)22 621 36 11
Therapist: Michael Spyrka
Email: info@allen-carr.pl
Website: www.allencarr.com

## POLAND – Alcohol sessions
Tel: +48 71 307 32 37
Therapist: Maciej Kramarz
Email: mk@allen-carr.com.pl
Website: www.allencarr.com

## PORTUGAL
### Oporto
Tel: +351 22 9958698
Therapist: Ria Slof
Email:
info@comodeixardefumar.com
Website: www.allencarr.com

## REPUBLIC OF IRELAND
### Dublin
Tel: +353 (0)1 499 9010
Therapists: Paul Melvin & Jim
McCreadie
Email: info@allencarr.ie
Website: www.allencarr.com

## ROMANIA
Tel: +40 (0)7321 3 8383
Therapist: Cristina Nichita
Email: raspunsuri@allencarr.ro
Website: www.allencarr.com

## RUSSIA
Allen Carr's Easyway to Stop
Smoking
Live Seminars & Online Video
Programme
Tel: +7 495 644 64 26
Freecall +7 (800) 250 6622
Therapist: Alexander Fomin
Email: info@allencarr.ru
Website: www.allencarr.com

Allen Carr's Easyway to Stop
Drinking
Live Seminars & Online Video
Programme

Tel: +8 (800) 302 80 68
+7 985 207 47 93
Therapist: Artem Kasyanov
Email: info@allencarrlife.ru
Website: www.allencarr.com

## St Petersburg
Please check website for details
Website: www.allencarr.com

## SERBIA
### Belgrade
Tel: +381 (0)11 308 8686
Email: office@allencarr.co.rs
Website: www.allencarr.com

## SINGAPORE
Tel: +65 62241450
Therapist: Pam Oei
Email: pam@allencarr.com.sg
Website: www.allencarr.com

## SLOVENIA
Tel: +386 (0)40 77 61 77
Therapist: Grega Sever
Email: easyway@easyway.si
Website: www.allencarr.com

## SOUTH AFRICA
Sessions held throughout South
Africa
National Booking Line:
0861 100 200
Head Office: 15 Draper Square,
Draper St, Claremont 7708, Cape
Town
Cape Town: Dr Charles Nel
Tel: +27 (0)21 851 5883
Mobile: 083 600 5555
Therapists: Dr Charles Nel,
Malcolm Robinson and Team
Email: easyway@allencarr.co.za
Website: www.allencarr.com

## SOUTH KOREA
**Seoul**
Tel: +82 (0)70 4227 1862
Therapist: Yousung Cha
Email: master@allencarr.co.kr
Website: www.allencarr.com

## SPAIN
Tel: +34 910 05 29 99
Therapist: Luis Loranca
Email: informes@AllenCarrOfficial.es
Website: www.allencarr.com

## SWEDEN
Tel: +46 70 695 6850
Therapists: Nina Ljungqvist,
Renée Johansson
Email: info@easyway.se
Website: www.allencarr.com

## SWITZERLAND
Sessions held throughout
Switzerland
Freephone: 0800RAUCHEN
(0800/728 2436)
Tel: +41 (0)52 383 3773
Fax: +41 (0)52 383 3774
Therapists: Cyrill Argast and Team
For sessions in Suisse Romand
and Svizzera Italiana:
Tel: 0800 386 387
Email: info@allen-carr.ch
Website: www.allencarr.com

## TURKEY
Sessions held throughout Turkey
Tel: +90 212 358 5307
Therapist: Emre Üstünuçar
Email: info@allencarr.com.tr
Website: www.allencarr.com

## UNITED ARAB EMIRATES
**Dubai and Abu Dhabi**
Tel: +97 56 693 4000
Therapist: Sadek El-Assaad
Email: info@AllenCarrEasyWay.me
Website: www.allencarr.com

# OTHER ALLEN CARR PUBLICATIONS

Allen Carr's revolutionary Easyway method is available in a wide variety of formats, including digitally as audiobooks and ebooks, and has been successfully applied to a broad range of subjects.

For more information about Easyway publications, please visit
**shop.allencarr.com**

Your Personal Stop Drinking Plan

The Easy Way to Control Alcohol

Allen Carr's Easy Way for Women to Quit Drinking

The Illustrated Easy Way to Stop Drinking

No More Hangovers

Allen Carr's Quit Smoking Boot Camp

The Easy Way to Quit Smoking

Your Personal Stop Smoking Plan

Stop Smoking with Allen Carr (with 70-minute audio CD)

The Illustrated Easy Way to Stop Smoking

Finally Free!

Smoking Sucks (Parent Guide with 16 page pull-out comic)

The Little Book of Quitting Smoking

Allen Carr's Easy Way for Women to Quit Smoking

How to Be a Happy Nonsmoker

The Only Way to Stop Smoking Permanently

Stop Smoking and Quit E-cigarettes

The Easy Way to Quit Vaping

No More Ashtrays

How to Stop Your Child Smoking

The Easy Way to Mindfulness

Smart Phone Dumb Phone

Good Sugar Bad Sugar

The Easy Way to Quit Sugar

The Easy Way to Quit Emotional Eating

Allan Carr's Easy Way for Women to Lose Weight

No More Diets

The Easy Way to Stop Gambling

No More Gambling

No More Worrying

Get Out of Debt Now

No More Debt

The Easy Way to Enjoy Flying

No More Fear of Flying

The Easy Way to Quit Caffeine

Burning Ambition

Packing It In The Easy Way
(the autobiography)

Easyway publications are also available as **audiobooks**.
Visit **shop.allencarr.com** to find out more.

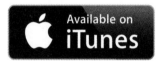
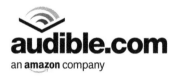